CW01667102

Recovering from Multiple Sclerosis

Real-Life Stories of Hope and Inspiration

George Jelinek
Karen Law

16
EasyRead Large

RHYW

Copyright Page from the Original Book

Published in 2013

Allen & Unwin
Sydney, Melbourne, Auckland, London

83 Alexander Street
Crows Nest NSW 2065
Australia
Phone: (61 2) 8425 0100
Fax: (61 2) 9906 2218
Email: info@allenandunwin.com
Web: www.allenandunwin.com

Cataloguing-in-Publication details are available from the National Library of Australia
www.trove.nla.gov.au

ISBN 978 1 74331 381 7

Set in 10.5/15 pt Cheltenham by Bookhouse, Sydney
Printed and bound in Australia by Griffin Press

10 9 8 7 6 5 4 3 2 1

MIX
Paper from responsible sources
FSC® C009448

The paper in this book is FSC® certified. FSC® promotes environmentally responsible, socially beneficial and economically viable management of the world's forests.

TABLE OF CONTENTS

'If you ever needed evidence that it IS possible to recover – yes RECOVER – from MS, you'll find it here in abundance. I hope this book will inspire everyone reading it to follow what these twelve people have done so successfully.'

Judy Graham, UK, author of Managing Multiple Sclerosis Naturally

'As a pediatrician who has been controlling his MS with diet for almost eighteen years, I wholeheartedly recommend this book for all people with MS. Diet and lifestyle changes offer enormous potential in facilitating recovery from this illness.'

Dr John Hovious MD, Bristol, Tennessee, USA

'Read this book and be inspired to regain your health, sense of invincibility and joy of living.'

Dr Heather King, GP, Auckland, NZ

'The stories are engaging, credible and highly readable. This book will be added to the "essential reading" for my own patients, whose stories mirror many of those told here.'

Dr Carole Hungerford, Sydney, Australia

'*Recovering from Multiple Sclerosis* offers real hope and incredible success stories of people around the world using nutrition and natural medicine-based approaches to treat MS naturally.'

James Colquhoun, filmmaker, USA: Food Matters *and* Hungry for Change

'It only has to be done once to show that it is possible. These stories confirm what I have seen with my own eyes. You can overcome MS. This book makes compelling reading for everyone with an interest in recovering from MS.'

Ian Gawler, Australia, author of You Can Conquer Cancer

www.overcomingms.org

ABOUT THE AUTHORS

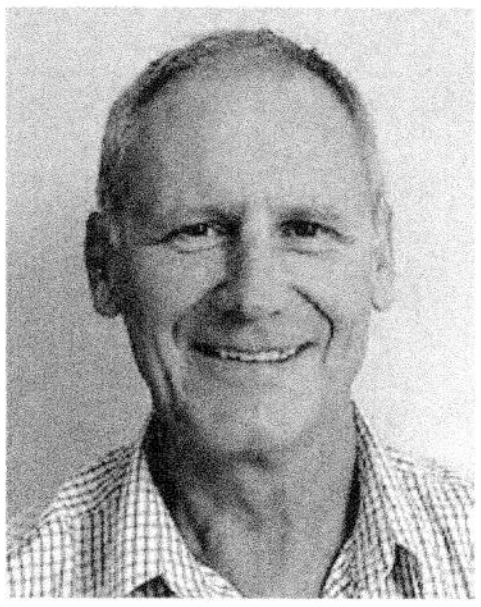

Professor George Jelinek is an emergency physician in Melbourne, Australia, with professorial appointments at the University of Melbourne and Monash University. He was the first Professor of Emergency Medicine in Australasia when appointed at the University of Western Australia in 1996, and is one of Australia's leading and most decorated emergency physicians, in 2003 being awarded the College Medal of the Australasian College for Emergency Medicine, its highest individual honour. George founded the international journal *Emergency Medicine Australasia* in 1989 and has edited it continuously since then, currently as Emeritus Editor. He has also written several major textbooks in emergency medicine.

In 1999, George was diagnosed with multiple sclerosis (MS), a disease his mother had died from 18 years earlier. He quickly researched the medical literature and realised that it was possible for him to stay well with intensive lifestyle change, which he adopted within weeks of diagnosis. Within months he had written his first book, *Taking Control of Multiple Sclerosis,* updated in 2010 as *Overcoming Multiple Sclerosis: An evidence-based guide to recovery.* In 2002 he began a series of live-in retreats for people with MS, leading these in Victoria, Western Australia, the Australian Capital Territory and New Zealand over subsequent years, with a retreat program in the United Kingdom starting in 2013. He started a website, *Taking Control of Multiple Sclerosis,* in 2008, revamping it as *Overcoming Multiple Sclerosis* in 2010. The website now has an active community of several thousand members. Overcoming Multiple Sclerosis UK was launched as a charitable trust in the United Kingdom in 2012, appointing its first Chief Executive Officer in the same year. In recognition of his work in multiple sclerosis and emergency medicine, George was a Western Australian Finalist for the 2008 Australian of the Year.

After a difficult year in 1999 with continuing disease activity, George stabilised his condition in 2000 and has remained well since, with no further relapses and no deterioration. Over a thousand people with MS have now experienced George's retreats and adopted his recommended lifestyle, along with the many thousands who have read his books, and hundreds of thousands who have visited the website. Many of these people have kept in touch with George over the years, including his co-author Karen Law. From the many who have reported recovery, George has chosen a dozen people for this book, with the aim of bringing hope to people everywhere that it really is possible to recover after a diagnosis of MS.

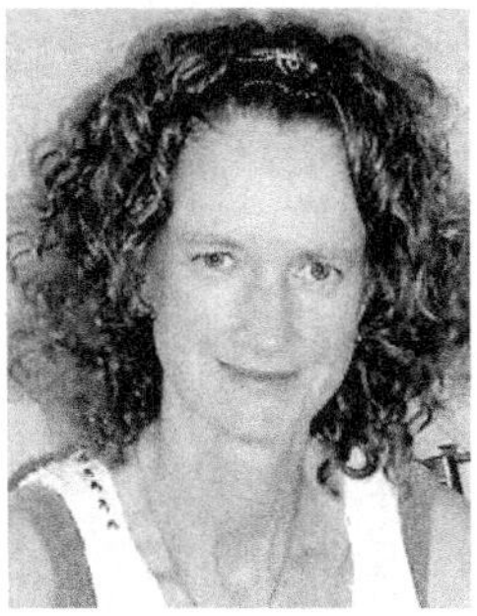

Karen Law is a writer, musician, teacher and mother of three, living in Queensland, Australia. She grew up in a village in rural England, and proceeded to a career in journalism, writing for an English newspaper. She and her husband migrated to Australia in 1995, travelling around the country for two years while Karen became serious about music, recording a CD and performing at folk music festivals. Later, after settling down and having children, she moved into freelance feature writing for magazines, specialising in parenting and the tourism trade. She has written scripts for ABC radio and released two CDs of her own songs, one for adults and one for children.

In 2003 Karen first developed symptoms of MS, which persisted and worsened until a formal diagnosis in 2010. Karen met George Jelinek soon afterwards. At the time she was in the middle of a spate of frightening relapses and was badly in need of hope. She found it. She also found the strength and courage to make major changes to her life, confront areas of emotional 'dis-ease', and get better. She sees her life very differently now, and her recovery as the result of a continuing process of self-exploration, discovery, and regaining balance. Karen strongly identifies with the spiritual aspects of healing, and acknowledges their importance in her own journey. Apart from her family, music has once again become the major passion in her life; she runs two music groups, teaches private students, and performs regularly. She has been free of MS relapses for over two years.

Helping to write this book is a symbol of the transformation that healing can bring; the realisation of a dream that would not have been possible before diagnosis. The twelve survivors profiled in this book, with their honest and courageous stories, have each also contributed to Karen's own recovery in a special way. Every time she listened to one of their real-life accounts, a little bit of inspiration and healing rubbed off on her—in the way that both she and George hope it also will for their readers.

FOR

Sandra, Sean, Michael, Pia, Ruby and Johnny

AND

David, Murray, Hazel and Roanna

FOREWORD

This is a book filled with the wisdom and experience of survivors. They are a source of information and inspiration from which we can all learn. My wife was diagnosed with multiple sclerosis over fifty years ago and is still sharing her love with me and showing how wrong doctors can be when predicting the future. We all have the potential to heal and outlive expectations if we are willing to participate in our life and health. We can learn from survivors and imitate them and let them and this book be our life coaches. When you heal and love your life and take responsibility, your body benefits.

George Jelinek and Karen Law have learned the same lessons I have learned from cancer patients. Self-induced healing is what we are all capable of. So read on; let the introduction, stories and concluding chapter be your guide and prepare you for life so you don't have to learn from a disaster, but let the experience of others help you to live up to your potential.

Bernie Siegel, MD

Author of *A Book of Miracles* and *Faith, Hope & Healing*

ACKNOWLEDGMENTS

We would like to thank Wendy, Jack, Keryn, Craig, Ginny, Carrie, Rebecca, Gaspar, Megan, Phil, Sam and Linda for their willingness to participate, their openness, their courage, and their honesty. We also thank our partners and family for their wonderful support and encouragement.

INTRODUCTION

Is it really possible to recover from multiple sclerosis? Open any textbook and the prognosis for people with MS is made all too stark. MS is an incurable neurological disease that is progressively disabling; the only thing that varies between people is the rate at which one becomes disabled. It is almost impossible to find the words 'multiple sclerosis' and 'recovery' in the same sentence in the medical literature or in a neurologist's office.

Yet the literature is remarkably consistent in documenting that genetic background influences only around a quarter of the risk of developing MS, and none of the risk of disease progression once diagnosed; the great majority of the risk is attributed to our environment, and most of these environmental influences are under our control. Saturated fat intake, omega-3 fatty acid consumption, sunlight exposure and vitamin D supplementation, cigarette smoking, response to stress, exercise, and many other modifiable risk factors have been shown in a variety of different scientific studies to influence the risk of developing MS as well as its progression. But the possibility of changing these risk factors is rarely mentioned to people with MS when they are diagnosed or when they attend their doctors for ongoing management. And the possibility of actual recovery is never mentioned. The best hope that is offered is delaying the inevitable.

For most people with MS, delaying the inevitable progression to disability is not good enough. Rather than accepting this prognosis, many of us with MS have chosen to make major changes to our lives, leaving no stone unturned in our quest to recover our health. We have chosen to do whatever it takes to stay or get well. The exact formula for doing that may vary between people, depending on their interpretation of the science behind these risk factors, but also on their understanding of themselves—not just their physical bodies, but their emotional and spiritual lives, and what 'dis-ease' or imbalance, if any, they may perceive as contributing to the illness.

We are fortunate to have had contact with many, many of these people from all over the world. In the age of the internet and social media, people actively trying to find ways of regaining their health after a diagnosis of serious illness tend to gravitate together. In general, these people are extremely positive, they have found hope, and they have faith that they can change their situations. They are careful about the language they use; they don't call themselves MS sufferers. We notice that unlike the major MS support and research organisations, they don't talk about cure, but rather healing.

A cure for MS seems to be a key focus of many of these MS organisations. But the notion of 'cure' implies the involvement of some external party working for years or decades to come up with something like a medication or procedure that can be applied to a passive patient, magically curing the patient's illness. Many research organisations are spending millions of dollars looking at molecules that target particular parts of the disease pathways in MS, or particular modes of therapy such as stem cells, which might be taken or injected or applied in some way to reverse the disease process. It is almost as if these organisations see MS as some kind of external invader, like a bacterium or virus that needs to exterminated.

But what of the more traditional notion of healing, where an individual understands MS as a fundamental internal imbalance, finds hope that getting better is possible, takes some control over the illness, makes internal and external changes—and, despite the prevailing paradigm of progressive disability, stays well, or even gets better and recovers function that had been lost? This is a vastly different experience for the person, even though the outcome of cure and healing may seem the same.

The experience is transformative. People change fundamentally; many find themselves on a journey more profound than merely regaining physical health. Many may confront difficult issues in their lives, seeing them as somehow being connected with the 'dis-ease' of having a serious incurable illness. Many start to wonder about the bigger questions we all face, involving the meaning of our lives, why we are here, and the impermanence of life. Some find that in the process of seeking to heal the illness, they begin to heal many other aspects of their emotional and spiritual lives, and their experience of life improves dramatically. Some even come to be thankful for a diagnosis that prompted them to follow this path.

Could this improvement represent recovery from the illness? 'Recovery' seems to be a significant omission from the lexicon of MS. Even with various types of serious cancer that very few people survive, such as pancreatic or bone cancer, recovery is still a possibility. There are unexpected survivors documented from most serious cancers, even when the cancer has spread significantly and would not normally be associated with survival. Indeed, at five years after the treatment of most common cancers, people would generally consider they had recovered. There are unexpected survivors of most serious illnesses, despite the worst of prognoses.

So why should recovery never be discussed in MS? We know people with MS who have gone decades without a relapse and with no discernible deterioration; in fact they are better than they were. Should they still feel that they could be struck down with paralysis, or worse, at any moment? How debilitating is it to have this constant possibility hanging over one's head? Surely we need to start talking about recovery as one of the genuinely possible outcomes from this illness.

While it is important to tell people about what risk factors they can change to stay or get well, and explain the science behind these recommendations so that people can have genuine hope that these changes can work (see www.overcomingms.org), we feel that it is equally important to present real-life stories of people who have made major changes and stayed well, or improved their situation. People who have actually recovered. This allows us to not only get a sense of what is possible, but to see and feel the texture of what recovery really looks and feels like. So that it is possible to see what it really takes, that not everyone does it the same way, that those who recover are not perfect or somehow extraordinary or different, that there are many roads to genuine health after a diagnosis of MS.

These are real-life stories of recovering from MS. We have chosen twelve people from among the many we know around the world who have recovered from MS—people of both genders and various ages, with varying levels of disability when they began this journey, and with different types of MS which they have had for different lengths of time. These are people who have chosen not to hide their illness or their outcomes after often difficult and challenging paths to recovery. We have interviewed them and written narratives that we hope reflect their unique paths through the illness and their lives.

Their stories are sometimes hard, sometimes ordinary, sometimes painful, but always hopeful and always inspirational. We hope their stories make the possibility of recovery more accessible, and break down the expectation of progressive deterioration after a diagnosis of MS.

A long, healthy and happy life is possible after a diagnosis of MS, and is within the reach of many people.

1

CALL OF THE KORIMAKO

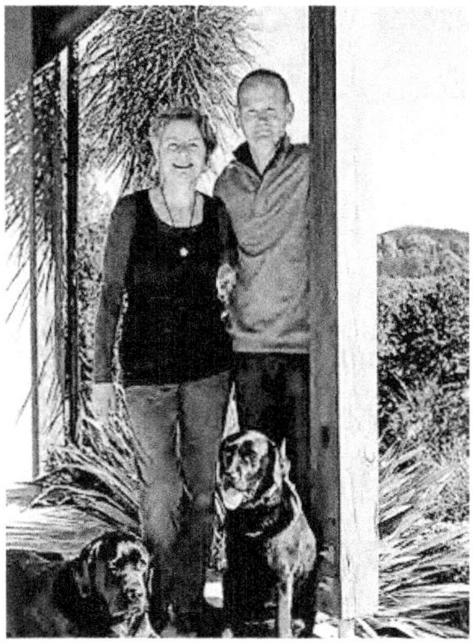

WENDY WOOD

Sitting on her timber balcony looking out over the magnificent Matakitaki River, Wendy Wood turned to her husband Steve in late 2009 and brought up the one subject that had been secretly haunting them both. Had the time come to leave their beloved guest lodge on New Zealand's South Island? Was multiple sclerosis about to take away their dream?

In fact MS had threatened to take away that dream before it had even begun. More than ten years earlier Wendy and Steve were living and working in Hamilton on the country's more populated North Island. Both originally from England, they had been attracted to

New Zealand by the active, outdoors lifestyle. When Steve's engineering employer relocated him there for two years they decided to stay for good, making regular fishing, walking and diving holidays part of their new lives. They were very happy in Hamilton, but the lure of the wilderness and beauty of nature kept tugging at their hearts. No longer content to live in the city and holiday in the wild, after a few years they had started making plans for a permanent move into the rugged countryside. They dreamed of opening up a guest lodge, a place where they could spend the next phase of their working lives. They were approaching 40, with no children, and the many years they had both spent working had given them enough spare capital to invest in 100 acres (40 hectares) of land.

During this period the tell-tale signs of MS had already started creeping into their lives. The first mild attack came after a hiking holiday with friends walking the beautiful Kepler Track. Wendy and Steve climbed high onto a mountain ridge, passing between Lakes Te Anau and Manapouri before descending the rough path on the other side. As always they carried all their food, clothes and camping gear on their backs, enjoying the strenuous exercise and the challenge of the walk. A few days after returning home to Hamilton, Wendy noticed that her feet had started to go numb. When the feeling spread up to her knees she consulted her GP about the problem. 'He was great,' she remembers. 'He always took me seriously and never fobbed me off.' He sent Wendy to an orthopaedic surgeon, suspecting she may have constriction in her spine. However, a CAT scan came back clear and a month or so later the numbness disappeared. 'My doctor said we'd keep an eye on it but not to worry.'

Then in late 1998 Wendy and Steve set off on another long trek, this time walking the Abel Tasman Track. Again they carried all their gear on their backs, enjoying the four-day hike along the rugged coastal paths. As they walked they talked about their future, the plans and dreams they had for the parcel of land they had bought in the Matakitaki valley. They thought up designs for lodges, discussed ideas for sustainable living, native tree planting and eco-friendly guest rooms. 'It was always in our minds that we were going to build a lodge; we had all these great plans and my health didn't feature in our thoughts at all,' says Wendy. But on the final day of the walk their planning and dreaming was brutally interrupted.

'Towards the end of the hike I started to get severe pain in the backs of my knees,' Wendy remembers. 'It got so bad that I couldn't carry my pack anymore and poor old Steve had to carry mine as well.' They completed the trek with Wendy hobbling her way painfully over the final kilometres, and Steve soldiering on with his own pack on his back and Wendy's pack strapped to his chest. By the time they emerged from the track Wendy was having difficulty straightening her legs.

At the emergency department of the local hospital, the doctor thought cysts might be causing the problem. At that stage Wendy didn't connect the two leg incidents, but when she returned home her feet started getting numb again and she went back to her own GP. This time he sent her to a neurologist, fearing Wendy had a tumour on her spine. After a fairly lengthy MRI she went back for her results on Christmas Eve. Steve went with her for support; they were both very worried about the prospect of cancer.

The neurologist looked up at Wendy from his chair in the consulting room and said, 'I'm very sorry to tell you that it's not cancer, it's MS.' Had it been a tumour, he explained, he would have been able to operate and fix the problem.

Wendy and Steve were speechless. They were relieved that it was not cancer, but really didn't know what to make of the shock diagnosis. Wendy had very little knowledge of MS, and until then she'd had no reason to investigate the disease. 'I knew it wasn't nice, but I knew it wasn't something that was going to kill me straight away,' she says. The neurologist referred Wendy to the local hospital for intravenous steroids, which were helpful as the numbness subsequently subsided. As he was not fully convinced it was MS, he also recommended getting a second opinion and referred Wendy to a leading MS specialist in Auckland.

'This second neurologist confirmed that I had MS, but he also told me it was quite likely that I had benign MS and might have no more difficulty than just occasional patches of numbness,' Wendy recalls.

'We talked about the disease and he told me there was no need to take drugs at this stage, but that steroids would help if there were any more episodes—and interestingly, he also recommended a "heart smart" diet.' He also quizzed Wendy on her medical history, looking for clues about past illnesses and infections that may have triggered the disease. Wendy remembered that a couple of years earlier Steve had contracted chickenpox and had been quite unwell for a time. After nursing him at home, Wendy had later developed shingles in a line across the small of her back. It was not the worst case of shingles, but bad enough to be uncomfortable. The neurologist certainly considered this significant, particularly as the MS lesions that had shown up on her MRI exactly mirrored the line of shingles on her back.

With a mild diagnosis of MS confirmed and discussed with her GP, Wendy went back to her former life, blissfully unaware of what the disease would have in store for her. She and Steve decided to put their plans to build a guest house on hold for a year, to see whether Wendy's health was going to be reliable. They carried on with their busy lives in Hamilton, staying in their jobs at one of New Zealand's biggest dairy companies, where Steve was a control engineer and Wendy was a business analyst. They continued hiking, though they chose to go on slightly shorter walks where they didn't need to carry quite as much equipment. And there were no more problems with Wendy's legs. Partway through the year they enjoyed a diving holiday, and again it was incident free. After twelve months, and firmly believing the benign prognosis, they decided to take the plunge and build their dream lodge. 'My health was really back to normal and I felt perfectly fine,' says Wendy. 'Steve and I sat down and had a real heart-to-heart about whether we should carry on with our plans. As I had been well for the whole year we decided to go for it.'

Their 100 acres at the top of South Island was steep, overlooking a beautiful river valley. Wendy and Steve identified a house site and set about planting around 4000 native shrubs and trees to attract birds and other wildlife. They did this themselves, taking time out from their busy working lives to clear, dig, plant and water the ground. The surroundings were breathtaking, and whenever they spent time in the Murchison area to tend their land they were reminded of why this move was so important to them. It was peaceful, nurturing, beautiful—part of the stunning wilderness that had convinced them to move permanently to New Zealand in the first place.

Throughout 2000 and 2001, their dream slowly began to take shape. The landscape was starting to flourish as the plants grew up around the house site. Wendy and Steve commissioned a local architect to turn their ideas into reality and create a haven for themselves and their future guests. The final lodge design was a timber construction over three levels that included three guest rooms, all with balconies overlooking the river valley. Upstairs, a communal north-facing deck joined the common lounge room. Three internal flights of stairs were needed to link Steve and Wendy's living quarters with the guest areas: it was a house designed for the environment, not for disability. And why shouldn't it be? Throughout this whole period of planting, designing and finally building their dream lodge, Wendy's health remained perfectly stable.

By mid 2001, the lodge was almost ready to open for business. The garden was establishing, the building was finished: all it needed was a name. One morning Wendy and Steve were in their kitchen in Hamilton, listening to their favourite radio program while getting ready for work. 'Just before the news each day they used to play a different bird call,' Wendy remembers. 'That day it was the korimako, the New Zealand bellbird. When they announced the name, Steve and I just looked at each other and knew that was what we were going to call the lodge,' she says.

The olive-green korimako, with its beautiful bell-like call, was just one of the many bird species that were becoming abundant around the lodge, attracted to the native garden Wendy and Steve had planted. The kea and kaka, both types of mountain parrot, were becoming frequent visitors too, as was the New Zealand falcon.

In 2001, Korimako opened for business for the first time. Wendy and Steve took guests all summer, watching their dream come to life after so many years of planning. Wendy loved the new lifestyle, the chance to plant her own vegetable garden and use the produce in the meals she cooked. And she loved sharing this wonderful bit of wilderness with the many visitors who arrived from all over the world. It sat easily with her friendly, open nature and passion for the environment.

For three years Wendy and Steve ran the lodge during the summer months, returning to Hamilton for contract work each winter. They continued with all their other outdoor activities too, skiing during the snow season, diving, fishing and hiking in the warmer months. Throughout this whole time there was not one single recurrence of the numbness or painful symptoms that had prompted Wendy's diagnosis in 1998. 'I knew that I had MS because I had been told that I did, but I didn't have any manifestations of the disease, apart from slight numbness in my fingers and toes,' she says. 'I didn't feel ill and I could do everything I wanted to do. I was thinking this idea that I had benign MS was probably right.'

In 2004 Wendy and Steve left Hamilton altogether and moved permanently into the lodge. They still only took guests in summer, but used the land all year round, grazing dairy cows on the spare acreage. They also acquired two gorgeous black labradors: Oscar—the lodge's official guest welcome officer—and Shadow.

Everything continued to run smoothly. By 2005 Wendy had been living with MS for around seven years, and in all that time had only had two fairly minor relapses. Then, imperceptibly at first, there began a very slow but steady slide into disability. This was something Wendy was totally unprepared for. Without any warning the disease had become progressive, and her physical and mental functions started to suffer. 'To begin with, things just felt a bit odd down my right side. It was hard to put my finger on anything specific, but I started to feel slightly unbalanced,' she remembers. 'Then a few months later I started to trip over. My balance was obviously getting worse and I developed foot-drop in my right foot.'

With these new and troubling symptoms to contend with, Wendy went to the local doctor's clinic for advice and was referred to the nearest neurologist. 'He just looked at me and said, "Well, you've got MS—what would you like me to do about it?", which was astonishing.'

So Wendy went back to the lodge with its three flights of stairs, its steep rocky paths and its vegetable garden built into the hillside. But as the months went by everything became harder and harder to manage. 'I began to get incredibly tired and I also started to have disturbed vision,' she recalls. 'Then I started wobbling, and once it started it just gradually got worse over time.' This wobbling came with a feeling that Wendy was literally walking on ice and needed to be careful where she put her feet.

Then the bladder control problems started. Wendy found she was constantly needing to locate toilets to avoid accidents whenever she went out. She managed the problem well, but it was affecting her quality of life. 'It was such a horrible symptom, like being a little girl again and needing reminders to go to the toilet all the time before leaving the house,' she recalls.

Her speech, memory and concentration also started to suffer. 'I found myself stumbling over my words and slurring my speech. That was very disturbing because it felt like I wouldn't even be able to hold a conversation anymore,' she says.

Weakness and clumsiness in her fingers meant she no longer enjoyed sewing, which had been a pleasurable hobby, and soon the vegetable garden became off-limits as well.

Other people, including guests at the lodge, were starting to notice Wendy's physical and cognitive problems. She managed to hide the full extent of her disability, but it was always Steve who carried platters of food from the kitchen, who poured wine, who served the meals. 'I had to tell guests that I had MS because they would see me tottering around and wonder what was wrong with me. I just dropped it into the conversation, but I always felt guilty burdening strangers with my problems.'

By 2009 Wendy was struggling to plan and cook a whole meal by herself, as the time spent standing up in the kitchen was causing terrible back pain. Her vision was often blurry and fatigue was a constant problem. 'I'm incredibly independent so I wouldn't let it stop me, but it was certainly very tough,' she admits.

By now she was stumbling a couple of times a day and falling flat on her face about once a week. 'If there was something there for me to trip over I would go completely flying and land on the floor. Luckily I never got badly hurt—except for my dignity,' she recalls.

'We were still running the lodge and I just had to carry on as best I could, but in the end we started to talk about selling up and moving somewhere flat that would be more suitable for me,' she admits. 'We kept putting off the decision because Korimako was our dream and we had been really happy there,' she says. But as Wendy's symptoms continued to worsen, the decision to leave seemed inevitable. 'I think Steve was finding me difficult to live with because I was getting angry at our situation.'

Known for being calm, logical and dependable, Wendy felt those traits were disappearing as she slid further into disability. 'The calmness was going because I was frightened, the logic was going because I was finding it difficult to reason, and I really wasn't dependable anymore because I wasn't sure I could follow through on anything,' she says.

In her sun-lit timber kitchen early one morning, Wendy was leaning against the workbench, gathering the strength she needed to prepare breakfast for the guests. The dawn chorus had been spectacular that day, and through the open window she could see the mountain ranges in the distance and hear the rush of the river over rocks where the trout would be hiding. Inside, the familiar sound of the radio interrupted Wendy's thoughts. She'd missed the morning bird call that day but the news had just finished and the presenter was announcing a guest—a medical professor from Australia who would be talking about MS.

Wendy's ears pricked up. She sat down on one of the big kitchen chairs to listen. 'When I heard Professor Jelinek talking that day, it was the first time I'd been exposed to the thought that there was anything any of us could do about MS,' she says. Over the next few days Wendy replayed the interview several times on her computer, letting the evidence-based recommendations about a low saturated-fat diet, vitamin D, exercise and meditation sink in.

'From the start I found the evidence very convincing. I went to see my local GP and I told her about what I had heard and that I was considering changing my diet,' Wendy says. 'She was very interested and it turned out she was a vegan herself, so had no concerns about the diet.' Her GP had also, as part of her medical training in Australia, been exposed to Ian Gawler's work on mind–body medicine. 'She loved the concept of empowering patients to take control of their own health,' Wendy says.

With a supportive GP and a growing belief that lifestyle change could help her recover from MS, Wendy set about altering her diet to fit in with Professor Jelinek's recommendations. Up to this point she had always believed she had eaten well. The vegetable garden at Korimako was flourishing with an abundance of garlic, tomatoes, broad beans, zucchini, rhubarb and potatoes. Free-range eggs came from the local farm and top-quality meat—wild and organic where possible—was reared on their land or sourced from the town butcher. Delicious chocolates and desserts were also part of the lodge's fine-dining experience, as well as platters of rich cheeses to complement an interesting wine list. While this constituted great cuisine, much of it did not comply with the Jelinek diet for MS and had to go. Wendy increased her vegetable intake, reduced meat considerably and removed dairy products from her diet altogether. She also decided to start supplementing with vitamin D, assisted by her supportive GP, quickly raising her levels above 150 nmol/L as suggested.

Just one month later she experienced a dramatic improvement in her MS symptoms. 'After just four weeks I found that my fatigue disappeared, and then my back pain went away as well,' she says with relief. 'These two things made such an enormous difference to my life; suddenly I was able to function properly again because I didn't have this overwhelming tiredness anymore. And I was able to stand up without being in pain.'

Her almost instant improvement was a huge incentive for Wendy to stick to the diet and keep her vitamin D levels up, which she did for the next two years. 'It really made me believe that there was something in this. I had nothing to lose and everything to gain; if this was going to help then I thought maybe we could stay living in our little piece of paradise for a bit longer.'

Wendy started keeping a diary of her MS symptoms, keen to chart the improvements as they occurred. She didn't have too long to wait. By February 2011, just one year after changing her diet, she listed a whole page of improvements in addition to the welcome disappearance of fatigue and pain. Firstly her balance was much better and she realised she had not fallen flat on her face for several months. She was sleeping more comfortably too, and had far greater energy levels during the day. Walking still required concentration, and foot-drop remained a problem, but now she could walk for a whole kilometre (over half a mile), slowly, with only a couple of rests. Her bladder function had improved, with slightly less urgency than before; sensation was returning to her hands and feet, which had been numb for years. Her memory and concentration were also sharper and she was able to enjoy reading again. 'Before that I used to start a book and then forget what had happened in the story when I picked it up again,' she recalls.

There were also some unexpected bonuses that had nothing to do with MS. Wendy noted with delight that her weight, which had risen to 72kg (160lb) in 2010 after three years of increasing disability, had now stabilised at 60kg (132lb)—the same weight she had been on her wedding day 25 years earlier. The terrible itchiness she had always felt in her skin had also vanished. 'I put that down to removing dairy from my diet, so that was an added incentive to stay off it,' she says. And for some reason her hair returned to the curls and ringlets of her teenage years, and her skin glowed.

One year later the improvements were still clocking up. By now her fingers and hands had lost their clumsiness, and for the first time in years Wendy was able to use pins, needles and scissors without dropping them. She could even thread a needle. Mentally her cognitive skills were improving too, and she could reason out a dressmaking pattern and complete sewing projects quickly and successfully. 'That was so great, especially as I had lost weight and needed to alter clothes to suit the new, slimmer me,' she laughs.

Her balance continued to improve, and for the first time she was able to stand on one leg while getting dressed. Yoga was helping her physical mobility and flexibility and she even progressed to shoulder-stands.

After years of letting Steve do all the serving at the lodge, Wendy found she could carry plates of food again without fearing she would drop or spill them. She was also enjoying the challenge of preparing complex meals for guests, cooking them and even clearing up afterwards.

Other people noticed the changes too. Wendy's physiotherapist, who had known her for years, commented, 'You're not slurring your speech anymore.'

Wendy started to feel socially confident again and far more optimistic about the future.

For a while, however, Wendy and Steve's lives at Korimako Lodge still seemed to be hanging in the balance. Since their first tentative discussion about finding a more suitable place to live, they had put the conversation on hold, waiting to see what changes the new lifestyle might bring. They were certainly very hopeful, and Wendy was markedly better both physically and mentally—but something stopped them from celebrating just yet and declaring a victory over MS.

In the end it took a residential MS retreat to really cement the belief that overcoming the condition was possible and allow Wendy to feel confident about the future. The retreat also reintroduced Wendy to meditation, and tightened her adherence to the whole diet and lifestyle package. 'I had been sticking to the diet 95 per cent for those first two years, but sometimes I would cheat,' Wendy says. 'Not because I couldn't resist certain foods but because I wanted to be polite in social situations.' After the retreat, she resolved never to knowingly eat saturated fat again, and she upped her daily intake of flaxseed oil. 'I left feeling completely empowered in my own health and not embarrassed over my diet any longer. I also started pursuing lots of different exercise options,' she says.

On her return, Wendy also booked in to see her supportive GP, keen to share her latest health insights. 'She was really pleased to see how much I had improved, and she even encouraged me to meditate,' says Wendy gratefully. 'When I got back from the retreat she gave me meditation lessons in the surgery. She'd book a double appointment for me and we'd sit cross-legged on her consulting-room floor and she'd talk me through a guided meditation,' Wendy says. 'Then we'd swap roles and I would talk her through one.'

As well as bringing a more mindful approach into daily life, the retreat also put Wendy in touch with her emotions in quite a profound way. Over the fourteen years she had been living with MS, through her initial diagnosis, early mild disease course and later disability, Wendy had never really allowed herself to grieve. She had felt anger, particularly when the disease became progressive and threatened her lifestyle, but she had never cried. 'On the last morning of the retreat I woke up in my room, which I shared with two other ladies, and I was sitting on my bed thinking about my life,' she remembers. 'Suddenly I just burst into tears—it was just bubbling up from inside me. I wasn't really distressed, but finally all this emotion was coming out,' she says.

Travelling back home on the plane, now in touch with this emotional side of her nature, Wendy resolved to tackle an area of unrest in her life. It was something that had been lying dormant since her childhood, growing up in the south of England. 'My relationship with my father had always been at arm's length,' Wendy admits. 'He was very buttoned-up emotionally, whereas my mother was far more demonstrative and open with her love.' Wendy says that when she was eleven, her father decided to move to Spain to pursue his career. The idea was that the rest of his family would join him there, but the reunion didn't happen. 'He actually lost contact with us. Three years later he suddenly returned because things hadn't worked out for him in Spain. I think I grew up a lot at that time, and it had a big impact on my relationship with him, though I kept my feelings hidden,' Wendy says.

Leaving the MS retreat all those years later, Wendy started drafting a letter to her father. He was still alive, aged 83, although her mother had died some years earlier. Wendy says the last she'd heard of her father was an email he'd sent her eight years earlier, giving her the news that he had remarried. She had lost touch with him since then. Now she decided it was time to attend to this unfinished business, to address the issues she still had with him and reopen communication once again. Three weeks later the letter was written and ready to be sent. As she dropped it into the mailbox she felt a sense of enormous relief, a real unburdening, as if bottled-up feelings of resentment were being released after nearly 40 years. 'A few weeks later I got a reply. Not an email but an actual letter. Now we are communicating again,' she says.

In October 2012, Wendy drew up yet another list of improvements to her MS symptoms. All the major benefits had stuck: the improved balance, lack of fatigue and pain, sharper cognitive ability and memory, and improved speech. In addition to all of these, Wendy was thankful for greatly improved bladder control, and a return of normal feeling to her hands and feet. She also found that she could climb up and down stairs with only minimal support. 'I actually think all the stairs at Korimako helped me because they kept me using my legs for longer,' she says. Wendy was able to walk on uneven ground without stumbling, and could now walk for one kilometre without needing to rest, with foot-drop no longer such a problem. Her vision was also back to normal—no longer blurry or disturbed—and her gait, or 'MS waddle', was far less noticeable. Afternoon naps were no longer needed as Wendy had plenty of energy to get through all the normal daily tasks. And thanks to regular yoga and pilates she was much more mobile and flexible.

With Wendy's health still gradually improving, and the lure of Korimako as strong as ever, Wendy and Steve eventually got round to finishing the conversation they had started back in 2009 when MS was threatening to destroy their dream. 'We finally sat down to discuss our situation, and Steve asked me what I reckoned we should do, whether I thought we needed to sell up,' recalls Wendy. 'I really didn't need to think about it at all. This place is so beautiful and there is nowhere else I would rather be.

'I am really optimistic that I am going to be well. I'm looking forward to being able to dig the vegetable garden again soon, and even go fishing and hiking again one day,' she says.

Every day, as she enjoys a gradual return to health, Wendy wakes up to the beautiful dawn chorus, the glorious mountain views, and the sound of the Matakitaki River flowing through the valley. And she is extremely thankful to still be there, in her own little piece of paradise.

2

THE HEALER

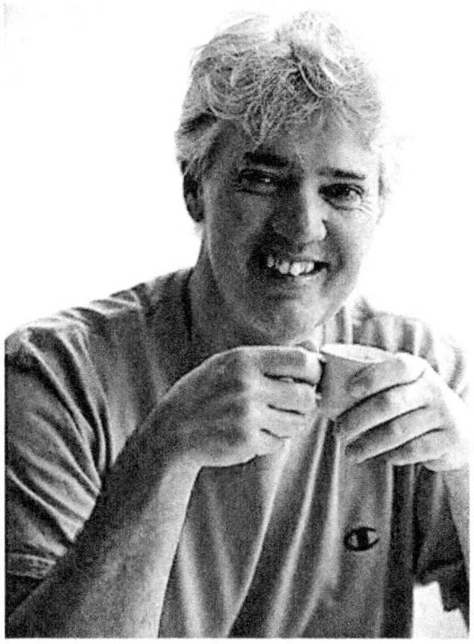

JACK MCNULTY

The head cage clicked shut, the table slid back, the radiologist left the room and suddenly Jack McNulty felt very alone. Well-travelled and confident, Jack was at ease in most situations, but here in this Zürich hospital, conversing in a foreign language, he was becoming agitated and very scared. His Swiss wife Silvia was in the waiting room, ready to take him home after the MRI. Back to their apartment in the city—to their busy, successful, agreeable life.

Lying inside the dome, Jack felt as if the machine was peering right inside him, stripping away his soul. He could remember one critical instruction from the technician—'don't move'—but it was becoming increasingly difficult to follow it. The tranquiliser he'd taken didn't seem to be working.

Jack tried to keep his eyes shut as the loud clicking noises began. Then the jackhammer started and he remembered another warning from the technician—'this will be loud'. The pounding continued and Jack started to feel tighter and more enclosed. He wanted to turn his head to make it more comfortable but, remembering the instructions he didn't dare move. With panic rising, the sheer volume of sound pulsated inside him and seemed to squeeze the air out of his lungs.

'Help,' he called out, sheepishly at first, 'I'm having some trouble—help.'

There was no response so he tried again, then louder, and in German. 'Bitte, bitte ... ich brauche hilfe.'

Still nothing happened, just the machine pounding and the feeling of panic rising in his chest. Then Jack remembered the emergency button that he was clutching in his now sweat-soaked hands. He pushed it. Nothing happened. Frantically he pushed it again. 'Help!' he cried out, then pushed the button again and waited ... pleaded and waited ... whimpered and waited.

Finally he was sliding out of the tunnel and a technician was apologising for the delay, removing the cage from his head and asking if he was okay. Jack sat up and drew as much air into his body as he could. He no longer cared about being abandoned inside the machine, nor did he berate the technicians who had left the room for a minute and missed his panic call. He was just relieved to be sitting upright again.

The slow response to his distress turned out to be something of a blessing. It meant that the first phase of the scan had completed successfully and wouldn't need to be repeated. As Jack sat there recovering from the ordeal, he felt the tranquiliser he'd taken earlier start to have an effect. By the time the technicians were ready to glide Jack back into the tunnel, the hammering sounds had become almost soothing, something to analyse rather than fear. In no time at all the room fell silent again and Jack was being eased out of the machine to return to his wife, the sunny street outside, their apartment. To wait for the news that would change his life completely.

That life had begun almost 50 years earlier. Born in Turkey to a Moroccan mother and an Irish-American father, he was the youngest of three children. When Jack was five the family moved to the United States—first to Oregon and then to Washington—and he had a typical American childhood. Mischievous as a kid, but never in serious trouble, Jack was very athletic and played a lot of sport. After high school he was offered the chance to play baseball at college level, but chose an academic scholarship instead. The baseball came to an end anyway with an arm injury after two years, but by then Jack was firmly on the path of the American Dream. He got a well-paid job in Silicon Valley—an exciting place to be in the 1980s and 90s—working in hi-tech telecommunications. He bought nice cars and lived in impressive houses, the last one overlooking the Golden Gate bridge. Then, at the age of 35, he turned his back on the whole thing to follow his own dream.

'Within my heart I just really wanted to cook. My mother was a very good cook and I had grown up eating really great, interesting food,' he says.

Jack decided to go to culinary school. He emptied his house of belongings, selling everything except a few personal items that fitted inside the boot of his car. 'It was a fabulous experience, very liberating. I'll never forget driving away and thinking that I could go anywhere. It was the ultimate freedom, I suppose.'

Two years later he was a qualified chef and had spent half that time on internships in Europe. He had also met Silvia, the Swiss wine educator who is now his wife. It was to Zürich that he moved at the end of his training, and in 2001 the couple married and later launched a cooking venture together, providing private catering and food and wine workshops for clients across Europe. Like most things in Jack's life, the business flourished.

In the summer of 2009, Jack and Silvia had just returned from a well-earned two-week holiday. Jack's brother and his family had been over from the States, and together the families spent time in Italy before cruising back up to the Swiss mountains. 'I remember feeling a bit dizzy when we were on top of a mountain in Switzerland, but I thought it was just the elevation,' says Jack.

Back home and with his mind once again on the business, Jack went for his customary jog around the streets of Zürich. He was dreaming up new ideas for his website, planning updates for his 'cooking with pumpkins' book, and thinking about developing the chocolate side of the business. It was a relatively long jog, which Jack often found useful for collecting his thoughts, but as he went over the top of a hill something disturbing happened to his right hip and knee. They just stopped working—or, rather, the messages he was sending from his brain stopped getting through. There was no pain and the feeling only lasted for a few seconds, but right from the start Jack was afraid. Over the years he had suffered many sporting injuries—pulled muscles, broken bones, sprains—but this was something different and far more sinister. He tried to come up with explanations—perhaps he hadn't stretched enough before the run—but those few strange seconds unsettled him.

The next day the vertigo started, coming in waves every hour or so, tossing his balance. With the vertigo came a return of the problem in his right knee and hip that had unsettled him so much on his run.

By the time he saw his GP the next day, he had more symptoms to add to the list: his right shoulder and arm had joined in the rebellion, and suddenly typing words on a keyboard or writing them down on paper was difficult. The doctor was unconcerned, thinking the symptoms were probably due to a virus, but referred him to a neurologist just to be sure. While waiting for that appointment Jack's condition deteriorated further. He felt cold and shivery—a creeping feeling that hugged his head, neck and shoulders—and a pressure settled on his neck, making breathing difficult when he lay down. His right leg and arm continued to periodically disobey orders from his brain, and occasional severe leg spasms sent a fire-like pain burning through his limbs.

Despite all these symptoms the neurologist agreed that a virus was the most likely cause of Jack's distress, though she did order an MRI to rule out anything nasty. Jack was convinced something serious was going on, but he wasn't sure how to tell his wife; her mother had been living with multiple sclerosis for many years and was doing very badly. In the end it was Silvia who was the first to admit what they were both thinking—that Jack might be heading in the same direction.

Walking away from the hospital after the claustrophobic MRI experience, Jack emerged into a sunny Zürich afternoon. Back at the flat, he spent the rest of the day faking normality while quietly worrying about the future. The next day he sat at his computer, in limbo, waiting to find out what was wrong.

'When the phone rang I knew right away it was the neurologist calling. I remember hearing her voice—professional but with a hint of alarm—asking if I could meet her as soon as possible.'

Jack felt a surge of anxiety but asked, in a surprisingly calm voice, if the news she had for him was bad. 'She told me the results of the MRI were nearly conclusive ... I had multiple sclerosis.'

Now the guessing game was over, Jack felt oddly relieved. His thoughts turned immediately to his older brother, with whom he'd recently shared a fantastic holiday. As a young man Charles had been handed a death sentence when he was diagnosed with stage three Hodgkin's disease. This type of cancer is usually fatal, but Charles opted for aggressive chemotherapy and managed to survive both the chemo and the cancer. Four years later the cancer returned. Again he chose to fight it and his prize was another year of life before the cancer returned for a third time. 'At that point most doctors tell you to tie up any loose ends because there's absolutely no hope,' says Jack. 'My brother's doctor refused to do that.' Instead he came up with another cocktail of chemotherapy and a new stem cell procedure. 'It came very close to killing him, but he managed to survive it, and he's now been clear of cancer for more than ten years.'

It wasn't only the story of survival against the odds that Jack was drawn to, but also his brother's attitude. 'He was always pushing boundaries. When Charles had his spleen removed he found out what the record was for getting out of hospital after the operation, and he broke it,' remembers Jack.

As kids growing up the brothers had always been competitive, urging each other on to new levels, but they were also good mates. 'I knew Charles had gone through all that and I knew it was in me to get over my situation too. It didn't feel totally under my control, but I knew I was going to do whatever I possibly could to climb that mountain.'

With these thoughts racing through his mind, Jack did something symbolic and important: he went out for a run. Silvia went with him, partly for physical support, but also as a joint display of strength; together they would take on MS.

'I had lots of incidents with my leg but I just slowed down, waited for it to pass and then carried on again,' Jack remembers.

Returning triumphant to the flat, Jack's stubborn streak took over. Just hours after receiving the diagnosis he sat himself down at his computer and started researching. Silvia sat next to him with her laptop, looking up all the sites in German while Jack scanned everything in English. Within an hour Jack had zoned in on the work of Dr Roy Swank, the neurologist whose patients had great success following a low saturated-fat diet. Silvia then discovered that some Swiss doctors were doing work along similar lines, researching dietary factors that might reduce inflammation.

This news brought some hope and gave Jack the courage to write down three goals: stop the relapse he was currently having, reduce or eliminate his symptoms, stop the disease from progressing. The next day when he and Silvia arrived at the neurologist's office to discuss his diagnosis, the list was firmly tucked into Jack's back pocket. They walked in feeling well prepared and almost aggressive. The neurologist, sensing this, spoke to them calmly and professionally, discussing Jack's symptoms and the evidence from the MRI scans. She pointed out 8–12 bright lesions in his brain and several other darker lesions. 'She explained that the bright ones represented new inflammation while the darker ones were old lesions, meaning I had actually had MS for some time,' says Jack. 'There was also a single lesion in my neck. This was new and medium-sized and was the cause of the problems I was having with my right leg and arm.'

The neurologist recommended steroid treatment for Jack's relapse and Rebif as a treatment to reduce future relapses. But she couldn't actually prescribe them until the diagnosis had been confirmed by a lumbar puncture.

This turned out to be a surreal experience more suited to a Monty Python sketch—or perhaps a horror movie—than real life. Jack still shudders to think of it.

'I was sitting upright, slightly bent over, ready for the first needle to enter my back. I remember the neurologist seeming really confident, as if this was something she was particularly good at.'

As the needle went in, Jack felt an excruciating pain explode inside his hip as the needle scraped a nerve. His blood pressure plummeted and he fell onto his side, temporarily stalling the procedure. 'Every time the doctor tried to get the needle in I felt a burst of electrical pain. It was too much for me, sweat was pouring off my face and in the end we aborted the whole thing.'

But respite was only brief. The next day Jack was back at the hospital, ready for round two. 'This time I was lying down, and a different doctor came in and told me there was an issue with my spine being curved the wrong way, but he wanted to have a try anyway.'

For the second time Jack felt excruciating pain shoot through his body. First one needle, then two, and then finally three were inserted. But the doctor couldn't get any fluid.

'I agreed that we would have one more try further up my spine. I was in tears but I just wanted the whole thing over and done with.'

At last, a sufficient amount of spinal fluid was collected, and Jack was allowed to lie on his side and recover from the ordeal. And that's when the farce began.

'It turned out that this fluid degrades if it is out of the body for too long, so it needed to be taken to the laboratory within an hour. The hospital hadn't booked a courier—they expected me to take the sample myself, and I was in no state to go anywhere.'

Jack had to lie down for half an hour while Silvia was summoned from the waiting room to be by his side. Finally they made their way out to the car, with Jack clutching the tube of precious fluid. 'Of course the laboratory was on the other side of Zürich, through lots of traffic. I was navigating and Silvia was driving as fast as she could, trying to beat the lights, switching lanes to get ahead. We just made it in time,' he remembers.

Now the lumbar puncture was completed, Jack had all the evidence he needed. A diagnosis of MS was confirmed and he was allowed to start treatment. With painful spasms, vertigo and loss of control in his limbs still causing big problems, he decided to tackle the first goal on his list: stopping the current relapse. And that meant steroid treatment. To begin with, the only effect this had was to make everything taste bitter—not nice for a chef. After two weeks with no change in his MS symptoms, Jack was getting impatient.

'I was concerned that the steroids weren't working. I'd given up running but I still went walking with Silvia every day and I noticed it was getting harder. I'd have two attacks every walk that would last for thirty seconds or so, and at night I was getting very painful spasms.

'I was sitting at my computer one morning writing an email to my neurologist, telling her about my situation and the fact that the steroids weren't helping,' remembers Jack. 'As I was writing I got up to make a cup of coffee and then it occurred to me that I actually hadn't had any symptoms that morning. No vertigo, no spasms and no loss of function in my limbs.'

Jack rushed off to find Silvia to share the news. 'We went for a walk straight away, and I did the whole four kilometres (two and a half miles) without a single incident. It still makes me cry now just thinking about it.'

Even though Jack's symptoms returned in the afternoon, that morning of respite gave him real hope. 'I'd gone a morning symptom-free, and to me that was a huge step.'

He never did send that email. That night Jack only had three spasms instead of ten, and over the next week the number dropped to only one major spasm a night, then finally to none. 'I chalked that up as my first victory,' Jack remembers.

With the relapse under control, Jack was ready to tackle the other goals on his list: eliminating all symptoms, and stopping the disease progression. While a fairly optimistic person, Jack nevertheless decided he would need some extra help to stay positive during such a challenging time. Right from the start he began surrounding himself with inspiring stories. Some of these stories came from books, some from the internet—examples of people who were overcoming disease in remarkable ways. He also turned to prayer and to the Bible, reading the scriptures for every reference to healing that might inspire his own journey. 'I typed up all these passages and read them as often as possible,' he says. 'Faith is very important to me and these quotations were really helpful because they are based on promises.' Jack's personal favourite comes from Jeremiah 30:17—*I will restore you to health and heal your wounds.* 'That is spoken very clearly and I hung on to those words,' he says.

Jack had every intention of allowing this spiritual side of healing to sit alongside the pharmaceutical methods being prescribed by his doctors. But it wasn't to be. The run of bad luck he'd had with medical procedures during diagnosis continued when he began taking medication. First there was Rebif, which went well for about two weeks, before taking a downwards spiral. 'I started with a low dose and that was fine, but as soon as I tried revving it up I got lots of side effects,' says Jack. 'Burning sensations that would intensify over 24 hours.'

He continued with the drug for several months, until one night he woke up feeling really depressed. 'That scared Silvia because she had read that one of the listed side effects was suicidal tendencies,' he remembers.

So Jack arranged to switch to Copaxone. Once again things did not run smoothly. 'The very first injection brought on a one-hour spasm in my leg and it was really painful, like the worst bee sting you could ever imagine.' Every injection brought pain, and after five days of this Jack realised that pharmaceutical drugs were not going to be part of his long-term healing package. Right after diagnosis this might have troubled him, but by now something else had given him a fresh burst of hope.

On Christmas morning 2009, four months after diagnosis, Jack woke up in his apartment to beautiful blue skies. Silvia was already at work, so he was alone. Staring out at the icy streets, he felt something stir inside him: he knew this was the day he would go jogging again. For the past couple of months he'd watched joggers enviously as they ran past him on his daily walks. Seeing them made him angry that MS had come into his life and taken away something precious. It also made him determined to run again one day, though he had no idea when. Now, on this Christmas morning, he did. It would happen immediately.

Jack was nervous and excited as he found some winter jogging clothes: long pants, two pairs of socks, a turtle neck, hat, jacket and running shoes. He stretched his arms and legs slowly, then collected his iPod and set it for shuffle before heading out the door. He was hoping to pass a neighbour on the way, someone who might offer a word of encouragement, but everything was quiet as he went down the stairs and out onto the freezing street below. As he reached the pavement Jack found himself conducting a quick mental body scan, something he'd never done before. His legs felt fine, his back was good, his neck felt a bit stiff but was okay. 'My mind kept telling me to simply head out nice and slow and see how far I could go. I was aiming for nothing, I just wanted to experience jogging again,' he says.

Setting out on what had been a regular running route, the first five minutes were all uphill. Jack jogged slower than in the past, but he was almost giddy when he reached the top with no pain and no symptoms. 'I remember feeling joyous and oblivious to the cold. I had already achieved a victory—anything else I accomplished that day would be a bonus,' he says.

Everything felt fine in his body, so Jack carried on. He was calm for the first time in months and he couldn't stop smiling. 'I'm sure I'd have looked very strange if I'd met anyone along the way, but the streets were completely empty,' he remembers.

Halfway along the route, when the road had flattened out and started descending, Jack became concerned in case his symptoms returned. He thought about stopping, but his legs kept running and he willed himself to carry on one step at a time. 'At one point I even closed my eyes and thought this must be what it's like to fly,' he recalls. 'I felt weightless for a fraction of time. It was an incredible feeling, but at the same time I wanted to feel my feet on the ground. I concentrated on my feet and felt them jar against the pavement.'

A few minutes later he knew he would complete the four kilometre circuit, but he sensed he was running too fast. His neck began to tingle and he kept repeating the mantra 'Go slow, go slow'. Finally he turned the last corner and stopped. Standing there, alone and triumphant, Jack became aware of the song that was playing on his iPod—'Healer', by Christian rock group Hillsong. 'I listened to the words of the song and simply cried,' he says. 'For the first time since my diagnosis I felt that I was going to recover. All my fears melted and I was left with an incredible sense of joy.'

The jog was more than a physical accomplishment; it was proof of something internal, something spiritual and private that Jack had been seeking for a long time.

'I truly felt God inside me on that day and I knew I would come out of this entire experience with a new purpose,' he says. 'That purpose is still mostly undefined but I know it's there.'

That run marked the start of Jack's athletic comeback, which continued slowly but surely over the next two years. Over time he increased his jogging distances. To start with his only goal was to regain the distance he'd been running before diagnosis. This was achieved after exactly a year, when he ran a six kilometre (three and three-quarter mile) route in 36 minutes. By March 2011 he was regularly running for half an hour twice a week, and in August that year he completed a 20 kilometre (twelve and a half mile) bike ride and a five kilometre (three mile) run. 'That was a big effort and it took me about a week to recover,' he remembers. Almost a year later Jack did a mini-triathlon: a ten kilometre (six mile) cycle, 3.5 kilometre (two mile) run and 300 metre (330 yard) swim. Shortly after that he climbed to the top of a very steep Swiss mountain.

Throughout this whole period Jack remained relapse-free, and his strength in the gym was constantly improving. 'At the start I could only lift limited amounts of weights, and certain exercises were completely off-limits, such as anything to do with my neck and shoulders,' Jack recalls. His legs were quite strong, so he worked on these while gradually building up stamina in the weaker parts of his body. In March 2011 he started working his neck and shoulders with weights. At first this was tough and made his body tingle, but Jack could sense his strength returning. Six months later these symptoms had gone. He went home and wrote in his journal, 'I no longer feel like the MS-guy at the gym,' and chalked it up as another victory.

By March 2012 he was up to 20kg (44lb) of weights for his neck, and some 30kg (66lb) for his shoulders. Three months later those weights had risen by another 5kg (11lb). 'I look forward to weight training because I get a real boost of energy that can last for a couple of days or more,' he says.

After the shock of diagnosis subsided Jack continued, with Silvia, to work hard at the cooking business.

As the months went by, food came to play an important role in his recovery. He'd already discovered Roy Swank within a few hours of diagnosis, and by January 2010 had studied Dr Swank's diet very closely. By this time he'd also found Professor George Jelinek's overview of all the MS research and was becoming convinced of the need to remove all saturated fat from his diet, as well as the need to supplement with vitamin D. The dietary changes could have been problematic for a chef, but Jack saw it as a challenge and an opportunity.

'Until then I had never paid any attention to nutrition; cooking was all about the taste, the flavours and the experience of eating,' he admits. 'But I actually felt like I had a headstart because I was used to looking at things from a food perspective,' he says.

Always using large amounts of butter, milk and cheese in his cooking, and with chocolate-making actually a part of the business, Jack had some serious work to do reinventing recipes. Silvia adopted the new diet too, both for support and because there was MS in her own family. To begin with they only changed their personal menus. Even so, there were some practical issues at work, particularly when it came to tasting the food Jack had cooked. 'When I make foods that don't belong in my diet I either taste and spit—so I don't actually consume the food—or I use Silvia as my mouth. She doesn't mind swallowing tiny amounts,' he says. If the taste of forbidden food on his tongue tempts him to actually start eating it, Jack uses a mental image as a warning. 'I picture myself in a wheelchair, and that takes any food urges away,' he says.

Since altering his diet, Jack's style of cooking has completely changed, and he sees this as a positive thing. His new methods have naturally spilled over into the business. 'I hadn't realised how much milk and cheese was in my diet before, but when I changed it was the greatest thing because it made cooking exciting again,' he recalls. 'Almost every cookbook is littered with traditional ways of cooking with eggs and dairy and I felt like this was a huge opportunity for me, not a penalty.'

Jack's new understanding about nutrition has created an ethical problem: he finds it hard when clients request dishes that he no longer considers healthy.

'At the moment I feel that the diet is *my* issue, and I don't want to force my beliefs on anyone,' he says, before adding, 'Let me rephrase that. I *do* want to force my beliefs on everyone, but I need to be careful about how I do that. For now I'm quite happy to cook something totally vegan for someone without them even realising it.'

On the business side, Jack took two months off work immediately after diagnosis, gradually increasing his hours as his health and fitness improved. A twelve-hour working day is not unusual for a chef, and Jack counts it as a victory that he can do that and stay well. 'I have a few minor symptoms that come and go. I can go for weeks without feeling anything, but I might wake up one day and my neck feels tingly. That's an indication that I'm getting tired, so I rest and usually by the next day I'm fine.'

With a real zest for life and enthusiasm that is totally contagious, Jack believes in celebrating all the little victories on the road to recovery. 'Progress is a series of little things, and whenever I achieve something I take a moment to appreciate it,' he reflects. The first time Jack walked up a big hill, worked a long shift in the kitchen or went running, he recorded it as a victory. 'I acknowledge these things to myself and I share my outbursts of enthusiasm with Silvia,' he says. 'And every year without a relapse is a big victory,' he adds triumphantly.

Jack records these events in his journal, something he started doing straight after diagnosis. 'I often look back to the same day a year ago, or two years ago, just to see how far I've come,' he says.

The past few years have been a time of growth and a time of change. Jack isn't glad that he has MS, and would not wish it on anyone, but paradoxically he also believes it's the best thing that's happened to him. 'MS has taken me to another level in my life, to the inner search,' he explains. 'In the past I was always staying within my boundaries, but this whole experience has given me enough faith to go that little bit beyond, and that is a great thing.'

Jack still writes in his journal, prays, meditates and exercises every day. And he still collects inspirational stories to surround himself with hope and positivity. Almost without realising it, he has become one of those stories himself.

3

RIDE ON FEARLESSLY

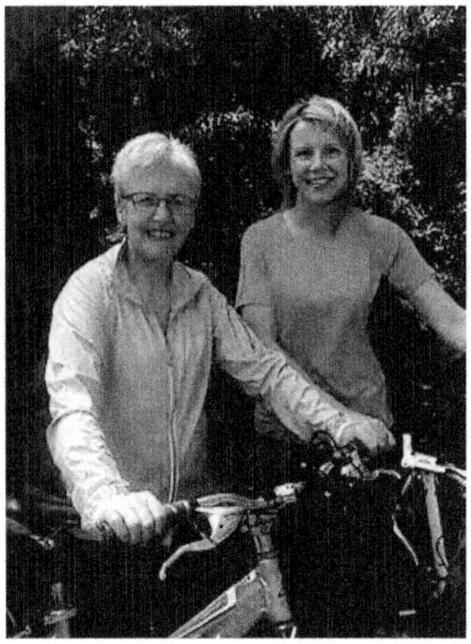

KERYN TAYLOR

Lake Hawea is a special place. Carved by glaciers and surrounded by mountains, it has a secret but stunning beauty. Keryn Taylor has spent part of every summer of her life by its tranquil shores. She has visited in winter too, when the mountains are capped with snow and the lake's already cool waters turn icy cold. Lake Hawea has wound itself like a vital thread through her life. 'It's a very quiet place and you can go down to the water and be the only person there,' she says. 'It's somewhere I've always gone for celebrations and happy times, but it's also somewhere I find myself going during difficult times.' In her 32 years she has known plenty of both.

Keryn was born in Dunedin, just a few hours drive from Lake Hawea on New Zealand's South Island. She grew up very happily with her mum and dad and older brother Mark. 'I feel I've been very much shaped by my family,' she says. 'I think of myself as a Taylor and I'm really close to both my parents and my brother.' Keryn's dad worked as an accountant and her mum stepped away from her teaching career to stay at home while the kids were young. A large, extended family added to the sense of community that surrounded Keryn as she grew up. Her granny, uncles, aunts and cousins all lived around Dunedin and were often part of day-to-day life, including holidays. 'Granny used to own a little house at Lake Hawea and I remember spending lots of family holidays there with my cousins. I've got loads of happy memories from that time, playing by the shore, riding bikes, boating on the lake, climbing up into the hills,' she says. In time Keryn's parents bought their own holiday house there as well, just a few doors down from Granny, and the tradition continued.

When Keryn started school she was noticed for being a bright student, but it was sport that dominated her life. And she was very good at that too, representing her district in team and individual events. When the time came to pick a high school, Keryn was keen to attend the one with the best hockey team. 'My mum and dad were pretty grounded though, and they suggested a co-educational school would be better, and how about the closest one,' she recalls. This turned out to be a great decision and Keryn's teenage years were filled with volleyball, basketball, hockey, sprinting, cross-country events and triathlons. 'I really played heaps of sports and I was pretty successful and won quite a lot of prizes. I used to love going away to sports tournaments,' she remembers. Keryn was a popular student; in her final year of high school she even became head girl. 'I was good at schoolwork, but I really saw myself as a sportsperson, and I think that's how other people saw me as well,' she says.

A professional sporting career would not have been out of the question. Keryn's dad had been a very good rugby player and family folklore says he broke his arm during his All Blacks trial. Keryn's brother Mark inherited the family sporting genes too, playing volleyball for New Zealand. But Keryn wasn't interested in pursuing sport as a career, either directly or indirectly. From a very young age there was actually something else she had set her heart on: she wanted to become a doctor. There were no other doctors in her extended family, and Keryn isn't sure where the idea came from. Perhaps it evolved out of the games she used to play with her doctor's set as a little girl. Or perhaps she was given the set because her interest in medicine was already obvious. Either way she spent many happy hours with a toy stethoscope round her neck and a white coat over her shoulders. 'I kept that little doctor's set for years and years,' she remembers. 'In the end my brother borrowed it for a fancy dress party and he lost it. I was gutted,' she laughs.

Keryn held on to the dream of becoming a doctor while she was growing up. However, turning the dream into reality required some serious effort. Medicine was highly competitive, and although she got straight As in her final year of school, this turned out not to be good enough. 'I was shown a graph of everyone's academic track record through high school. I saw the grades of people who got accepted for medical school and mine were way off the bottom,' she says.

Keryn didn't give up on the dream, although she did have to alter her method of achieving it. She applied to study physiology and psychology at Otago University and got offered a place straight away. She still played sport, but put more emphasis on her studies. At the end of three years she graduated with top grades and was finally offered a coveted place to study medicine. And so she started again, almost at the beginning of a six-year medical degree. It was a long and arduous path to take but Keryn never regretted it. 'I absolutely loved it. When I finally got to study medicine it was like Christmas for me,' she says. 'It kept getting better and better the more clinical work I got to do.'

Two years of lectures and book work were followed by three more years of clinical practice. Along the way she was presented with a real stethoscope, replacing the long-lost childhood toy. 'When I first got my stethoscope in medical school I called in at home and asked Dad if I could listen to his heart,' Keryn remembers. Just like she had done as a child, Keryn popped the scope in her ears and pressed the other end to her dad's chest. Nothing happened. 'I thought maybe he had that rare condition where your heart is on the other side of your chest, but there was no heartbeat on that side either,' she says. 'In the end I realised that I had forgotten to turn the stethoscope on!' she laughs.

By 2005 Keryn knew her way around not just a stethoscope, but a huge range of specialised medical equipment as well. She was on top of the science, the research and the human aspects of the training. Her success at medical school had proven to everyone that she was right to be following this career path.

She had managed to keep things in balance with a combination of sport and an active social life as well. Living with friends, she was in a serious long-term relationship, yet still maintained the strong family support network of her childhood. At the age of 25 Keryn Taylor was ready to launch herself into the world.

'I'd taken my final exams and started my year as a trainee intern working alongside first-year doctors to gain more experience,' she says. 'I was pretty excited at where I was headed. I was right on the verge of achieving what I had been working towards for so long,' she says. 'I was about to become a doctor.'

Part of her clinical practice midway through the year involved a six-week stint in the oncology ward. Keryn found that difficult, particularly when she discovered she knew two of the patients diagnosed with cancer. She had just moved on to a new job in orthopaedics when she woke up one morning with a funny feeling in her right hand. It was an odd sensation, a slight numbness—nothing major or immediately worrying. Keryn had never had any health problems and there was no history of MS in her family, so she didn't pay too much attention to it at first. But over a week, the feelings worsened. First the pins and needles started, then a bad sunburn sensation on her skin. Sharp pains went through her hand and arm whenever anything brushed against them. She could no longer open her front door and soon realised that she wouldn't be able to write when she started her shift on Monday morning.

'I got Mum to drive me to the hospital to get it checked out. They said it was probably a pinched nerve, but ordered an MRI anyway,' she remembers. The MRI was unpleasant, but not because she was concerned about what it might uncover. It was just that she'd never been inside one of those machines before and the loud, thumping noise started to overtake her. Keryn closed her eyes and imagined she was at Lake Hawea, staring into its clear waters.

The image comforted her until the procedure was over.

The next day she was waiting in the neurology ward when her scan results finally came through. A young doctor, realising who they were for, handed them to Keryn. 'I opened it up right on the spot to see the report, and I remember standing there outside the doctors' station reading the words "demyelination" and "lesions" and realising they were talking about me. It was totally unexpected and just the biggest shock I could possibly have imagined.'

Standing there on the verge of achieving her life-time goal, Keryn's whole world came to a complete stop. Independence turned to isolation, confidence crumpled and gave way to absolute terror. She stood there frozen, report in hand, as doctors hurried past her on their ward rounds. When she felt able to move again she phoned her mum and dad and asked them to come in and meet her at the hospital. 'Telling them was one of the most horrible things I have ever had to do,' she admits. But at least it meant she had some family support as she sat in the neurologist's office a few hours later and listened as he gave the official diagnosis of multiple sclerosis. The MRI had revealed a number of older lesions on her brain, and a much more recent and very active lesion on her spine. 'I was totally overwhelmed at that time. I was 25 years old and my whole life was waiting for me. I couldn't quite believe what was happening.'

Right from the start, Keryn was urged to keep the diagnosis secret. 'My neurologist and several senior colleagues told me not to disclose it because I would be discriminated against in my career,' she says. Already understanding that MS was going to have a huge impact on her future, this need for secrecy increased the fear. Keryn's thoughts quickly turned to her career. 'It seems ridiculous now but I remember asking the neurologist if I would still be able to work as a doctor,' she says. His response was not very optimistic. 'He said he knew of one doctor with MS and she was able to work as a part-time GP, so perhaps I would be able to do that.'

That was not what Keryn had been planning to do with her medical training. The neurologist's words kept churning round in her head later as she lay in the hospital bed receiving intravenous steroids. 'Mum and Dad were really upset by what was happening to me and I felt like I was a burden on everyone,' she recalls. Her boyfriend also came to visit her in hospital and Keryn could see that he found the news really hard to take in. Around this time their relationship, which was already troubled, ended.

Keryn told virtually no-one about the diagnosis. Worse than the fear of discrimination was the thought that someone might pity her. 'I didn't tell anyone and I tried hard to keep going. I thought if I could just manage to become a doctor then everything would still be okay,' she admits.

It was a difficult time and Keryn leaned strongly on her family. She moved back into her parents' house, where their love, support and practical help enabled her to get through the weeks that followed. The symptoms in her hands were starting to settle, but soon she had a new nightmare to contend with. Prescribed interferon to reduce further relapses, Keryn started to experience severe side effects to the drug. 'I was vomiting and I got ulcers in my mouth. Looking back, I'm sure that was a reaction to the stress as well,' she says. 'Psychologically it was hard to be injecting myself with something that made me feel so sick. I really felt lost and I was struggling to keep up with my studies because I was feeling so tired and run-down.'

Terrified of what would happen if she had another relapse, Keryn stuck to the interferon and did her best to cope. Her neurologist even put her back on steroids to try to reduce the side effects. All of this was hard enough to handle at home, but Keryn also chose to stay at work, just telling one best friend from medical school about her situation. The shifts were long and hard, and worse still her three-month elective training was just about to start. 'I had arranged to study obstetrics in London and then work with the anti-doping team in Montreal for the 2005 World Aquatic Championships,' she says. 'My neurologist recommended not going, and the Dean of Medical School said perhaps I should swap my elective block and do it in Dunedin instead,' she recalls.

Keryn ignored their advice. She set off for London with her secret diagnosis and her packs of interferon that had to be kept cold on the flight. And somehow she got through those three months despite fatigue, nausea and an overwhelming sense of fear that she would wake up one morning to find part of her body had stopped working. 'Luckily my brother Mark was in London at the time and he knew what was going on for me. Otherwise I'm not sure how I would have got through it,' she admits. 'It was very tough, but I also managed some fantastic travelling and it was amazing to spend time with my brother,' she says.

By the end of the year Keryn had made it back to Dunedin. Far from the triumphant celebration at the end of eight years of study, the successful completion of her medical training brought more relief than joy. Quietly Keryn Taylor became a doctor and started working at Dunedin hospital. She kept her diagnosis to herself, secretly living with the injections, the side effects and the fear. 'A lot of things shaped my initial view of how I perceived MS,' she says. 'It was always in the background and I continued to see people with progressive MS at the hospital, those who were having real difficulties. I had a very terrifying view of what my future was going to be like,' she remembers. 'I was just so frightened and it felt like there wasn't anything I could do. And I was so tired and sick with the interferon that I couldn't figure out if it was MS or a side effect or just because I was so anxious,' she admits.

Keryn's first position as a junior doctor was in psychiatry, and part of her on-call work covered the neurological ward. Just five months earlier she had been at the receiving end of treatment in that ward; the memory sat heavily on her mind. 'I just kept on working so that I wouldn't need to deal with my fears. I thought if I could hold that part of my life together I'd be able to keep going.'

It was around this time that Keryn wandered into a little bookshop in Dunedin after work one day. She wasn't looking for anything in particular, but an interesting title caught her eye and she bought a copy and took it home. She was still living at her parents' house, the childhood home that continued to provide a safe haven for her. It was here, curled up in a familiar armchair, that she opened the cover of Professor George Jelinek's *Taking Control of Multiple Sclerosis* and realised for the first time that she could do something about her situation. She could reclaim her life and potentially recover.

'It all made so much sense to me—the medical credibility and the importance of your emotions on your life,' she says. Almost immediately Keryn's single-mindedness took over and she decided to throw herself into the suggested lifestyle changes. 'My nature is that when I find something that I want to do, I just do it all the way,' she says. Keryn's mum adopted a far more cautious attitude about the book, suggesting that they try one or two things to see what worked. But Keryn was adamant: it was all or nothing.

She booked into an MS retreat in 2006. Her mum Joan went with her for support, a continuation of the family love that had surrounded Keryn for so long. The week was confronting for many reasons. Firstly because Keryn was not used to being open about her diagnosis, and here she was standing up and being counted as a person with MS. Secondly, she still harboured a lot of anger. At the start this seemed to be directed at particular people, but during the week Keryn came to see it differently. 'When I was at the retreat we had been learning about trying to let go of anger,' she remembers. 'The facilitator described anger as a hot coal that you want to throw at someone but which ends up burning your own hand instead,' she says. 'I remember talking to another participant during the break and she suggested that I might not just be angry at people in my past, I might be angry about having MS,' Keryn says. 'I knew she was right and that a big part of my healing was letting go of that anger and moving on.'

Joan Taylor had some healing of her own to do during the retreat. 'I'd never seen Mum upset before about the fact that I had MS,' Keryn recalls. 'She is such a kind and chatty person and I hadn't seen her fears exposed. I have always had a great relationship with Mum, but going through this together was really incredible,' she adds.

When Keryn returned home to Dunedin, back to her ward rounds at the hospital, back to her secretive life with MS, she found that a little bit of the terror had started to lift. Paralysing fear was at that time her main MS symptom, most of her other problems being side effects of the interferon. Keryn had switched to a second type of interferon, but it was only after she changed to Copaxone that she was able to get rid of the crippling side effects. 'It was such a relief and I was able to start running again,' she says. 'I hadn't been exercising at all until then because I felt so tired and sick all the time.'

Her typical Kiwi diet, high in dairy, meat and chocolate, needed some serious adjustment, and her vitamin D levels also needed raising. These two aspects were easily incorporated into her new lifestyle. Stress management, however, required a little more effort. 'I had pushed myself pretty hard for a long time wanting to study medicine,' she explains. 'Leading up to the relapse, things had been stressful working on the oncology ward and also in my relationship.' In the past Keryn had used sport as a way of alleviating stress. Now she started to incorporate mindfulness meditation into her daily routine as well. 'I think stress management is the final frontier for me. I'm still trying to find ways of improving my meditation rather than exercising at 110 per cent as my way of coping,' she says.

One particular healing meditation became significant for Keryn. With an image of the moon rising over Lake Hawea fixed in her mind, she imagined healing light pouring from the white sphere and entering her body, cleansing it of all disease.

As Keryn started to feel more hopeful about the future, Lake Hawea, with its tranquil surroundings and comforting history, wound its way into her recovery in another special way. Like countless times before she was staying at the family's favourite holiday spot with her mum and dad. 'The mountains, hills and lake were as beautiful as ever. You just knew they'd been there for all of time and any worries you had were just passing,' she says. Keryn was enjoying the serenity, beginning to feel more at ease with her situation. Joan encouraged Keryn to join her for a bike ride. The day was cloudy and slightly windy, but quite spectacular. 'We set out together and we must have had a tail wind all the way across the lake,' Keryn remembers. 'After an hour we stopped riding and realised we were at the very farthest point from the house.' The pair turned around and set off on the ride back home, but as they did so a strong headwind rose to greet them. Then it started raining, very heavily. Keryn's first instinct was to head straight for a cafe for shelter, or hide beneath a tree. But Joan had other ideas. She looked across at her daughter with a determined glint in her eye and said with bravado, 'Keryn, let's Ride On Fearlessly.' They rode all the way home in the pouring rain, braving the elements together. From that day on the phrase 'Ride On Fearlessly' became a symbolic catchphrase between mother and daughter, a sign of determination and confidence about the future. 'Mum often puts a little ROF in the corner of a postcard, or sends me a text with it on as a reminder,' Keryn laughs.

After starting work as a junior doctor in late 2005, Keryn worked her way through rotations in different areas of medicine at Dunedin Hospital. She finished psychiatry and moved on to obstetrics and gynaecology, which she also enjoyed. She was gradually starting to feel more sure of her future, both in terms of her health and her medical career. 'I got offered a more senior position with the obstetrics and gynaecology service, but it was a lot of high-pressure on-call work, and very unpredictable,' she says. By this stage Keryn felt able to live on her own again and moved out of her parents' house and into an apartment. She even felt strong enough to apply for work in England, but the medical borders had just been closed to New Zealand doctors, so she went there for a holiday instead. With every month that passed without a relapse, her confidence increased. 'When I arrived back in New Zealand I wasn't sure what to do so I took a psychiatry locum job in Wellington. I was pretty excited to be living independently again; moving away from Dunedin was a big step for me,' she recalls. When Keryn was offered a position on the training program for psychiatry she decided to take it. 'I loved the fact that in psychiatry you get to know people and spend time with them. I was really happy that I'd found what I wanted to specialise in.'

Living on her own, working successfully in a job she loved, connected to friends and family, the horror she had felt at diagnosis continued to fade into the background.

As the months turned to years, and Keryn stayed relapse-free, she became more open about her diagnosis. 'By 2010 things were getting a lot better and I was getting more and more confident about having MS. I wasn't thinking about it all the time and it wasn't such a big deal. One of my friends had been having a really difficult time and I always used that as the reason for not telling her,' she says. 'When I finally talked about MS she was so pleased I'd told her. She said it would have been nice to know that someone else was struggling as well as her.' As Keryn told more people, she realised that no-one felt sorry for her and that she wasn't a burden to anyone. 'There were a couple of people who were negative, but that was in a work setting and I realised that it was more their issue than mine,' she says.

Telling friends and extended family members was one thing, but telling potential boyfriends was another. 'My brother told me that when I found the right guy MS wouldn't matter to him. I didn't believe him at the time,' she remembers.

But he was right. In 2011 Keryn started dating a surgeon she'd known for several years. 'In the past when I told guys about MS it hadn't gone so well. But with Kush it was different. He is really proud of me and he sees it as a strength, not a weakness. I think it's wonderful to have met someone who feels that way about MS because it has taken me a long time to see it like that myself,' she says.

The year 2011 was significant in other ways as well. It was the year Keryn sat for her final psychiatry exams, passing them first time. 'Sitting those exams was a massive event in my life and all consuming,' she recalls. 'I credit the diet and lifestyle with my results, and I'm delighted to say that MS played no part in that year at all.' Leading up to the exams, Keryn was studying closely with medic friends who knew about her MS-friendly diet. 'I spent a lot of time with three other doctors and I got a reputation for being a bit of a health freak,' she says. 'In our study sessions I used to bring in juices and broccoli soup. If someone had taken chips into the study group it would have been like trying to smuggle crack cocaine into the library,' she laughs.

There is a serious side to her fanaticism too. In the last few years Keryn has noticed many friends and family members starting to live more healthily as well—notably her mum Joan. 'Seeing Mum change her diet and lifestyle has been wonderful,' Keryn says. 'Over the years Mum and I have done a lot of walking together, and she has really taken to it quite seriously,' says Keryn. Previously known as the non-sporting member of the Taylor clan, Joan is now a medal winner in her own right. 'Two years ago Mum entered the Masters Games in New Zealand and won two silver medals for long-distance walking,' Keryn says. 'The next time the games were held she entered again and won double gold.'

With her exams behind her, Keryn then secured a sought-after post in consultation liaison psychiatry and began two more years of work-based specialist training. This narrow branch of medicine focuses on people's physical and mental health, including the psychological reaction to having a physical illness. 'I really felt drawn to this,' says Keryn. 'I know what it's like to face physical health problems at a very young age. I hope that gives me empathy with people who feel real fear and uncertainty.'

Keryn is also conducting research into medication, lifestyle factors, depression and anxiety for people with MS. 'I really feel like my journey as a doctor has come full circle,' she adds.

Seven years on from diagnosis, and with no relapses in all that time, Keryn Taylor finds it hard to believe how she once felt about multiple sclerosis. 'To begin with I couldn't even say those words out loud and I was terrified of the future,' she remembers. 'It was such a difficult time in my life and I thought MS would take everything away from me—my physical identity and my intelligence,' she says. 'I didn't realise that it was already taking away the positive and happy person that I was.'

Today that positive outlook has definitely returned, though it is now tinged with a little reflective wisdom. 'I'm confident that I have overcome MS, but I really see that life is full of challenges. There will be times when I feel confident, strong and on top of the world, and other times when I won't,' she says.

And when challenges appear, Keryn will remember that bike ride with her mum at Lake Hawea, lift her head to the sky and ride on fearlessly.

4

WHERE HOPE BEGAN

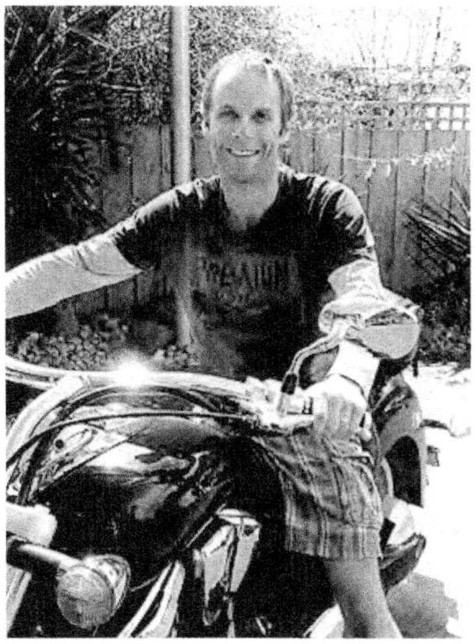

CRAIG WHEELER

Craig Wheeler has just one way to describe his life before he took control of his health. 'It was shit-ful,' he says.

The 42-year-old former marathon runner and ironman contestant doesn't mince his words. And why should he? In the space of just four years multiple sclerosis totally ravaged his body, costing him his physical fitness, his job and his marriage. By 2006 he was finding it impossible to be positive about a future that seemed likely to end in a nursing home. Soon.

Craig grew up in Leopold near Geelong, in Victoria, Australia. Born with his umbilical cord around his neck, his birth was dramatic and his life hung briefly in the balance. However, the trauma was soon in the past and he grew up healthy and strong. One of five children with a large extended family all living nearby, Craig had a reputation for being very athletic. He was keen on sport right from the start, and was very good at it. He played Aussie Rules football until he was about sixteen and showed enough talent to be invited to train with the Geelong Football Club, but a ligament injury in his knee steered him towards surfing instead. 'I started surfing when I was fifteen. Mum and Dad wanted me to do it properly and safely, as part of a club, so I joined the local surf lifesavers,' he remembers. 'When my knee got injured I decided not to have an operation because other people hadn't recovered too well from it. I just put my energy into surfing instead.' All his spare time was spent in the water, or training on the beach. In his late teens he also spent his Friday and Saturday nights partying with his mates. But he kept on top of his fitness and never got into drugs. 'That quite surprises me, because I was a bit of a loser as a teenager,' he admits. 'But I was always dead against drugs of any kind.'

Since it was sport, not study, that inspired him, Craig quit school as soon as he could. At the age of sixteen he began a five-year apprenticeship as a cabinetmaker in the family business. From 8a.m. to 4p.m., five days a week, he worked hard with his hands, learning the skills needed to make kitchen benches and cupboards. Before and after work he'd be running along the beach, building his strength and stamina before racing into the water for a surf. By the end of his apprenticeship he had started competing in the Australian Ironman Surf Lifesaving competitions, a beach-based test of strength, fitness and athletic ability. 'I had no swimming background so I had to start training really hard for that. Every morning I'd be down in the water,' he remembers. 'There are eight or nine competitions over the summer and I'd usually finish somewhere in the middle of the pack. I put a lot of pressure on myself as a competitor so I never really enjoyed it as much as I could have done, but I was definitely very fit,' he says.

Throughout his twenties Craig showed no signs of slowing down, continuing to work hard and train hard. He added marathon running to his list of achievements, clocking up very respectable times in the Melbourne Marathon two years in a row.

Meanwhile the family business that Craig's dad had been running for around 30 years was also keeping him very busy. With his apprenticeship completed Craig was now a fully qualified cabinetmaker, and at the age of 24 he also became a financial partner in the business. 'It was already an established, successful company and I was going into it with my dad. Still, we were both working 75 hours a week to get the jobs done,' he says.

It was at this time that he met Deb, his first wife; their son Jonah was born in the middle of 2002. Exactly six weeks later, Craig started getting severe double vision in both eyes. 'I could still see outlines of things but I was struggling to make out what I was looking at,' he recalls. He went to his GP and was given eye drops, which failed to solve the problem. 'Then my balance started to go on me,' says Craig. 'I'd fall over for no apparent reason and I often felt very dizzy and the room seemed to be spinning.'

Very worried by now he returned to his doctor, who referred him to a specialist. 'I was sent to a neurologist, and he was concerned about multiple sclerosis, so he sent me to one of the best MS neurologists in Australia,' says Craig. 'I had MRI scans and a lumbar puncture to try and find out what was going on.' The scans showed up evidence of a childhood stroke, which could have happened during Craig's difficult birth, but no signs of MS at all. 'The neurologist told me it didn't look like MS. He said I should go off and enjoy my life, which is what I tried to do,' he recalls.

Craig's enjoyment was short-lived. Just two months later, and with his eyes still causing him trouble, he started getting unpleasant sensations in his feet. 'To begin with it felt like I was walking on rolled-up ropes. Then the strange feelings travelled up my legs and I ended up losing power,' he remembers. 'I was standing beside my car one day and I just fell over straight onto the ground.' Over the course of that day Craig became almost paralysed. 'It never quite got to the point that I couldn't move at all, but I remember lying on my bedroom floor crying my eyes out and thinking I'd never be able to walk again,' he says. Craig was taken to hospital, where he had a catheter inserted to help him pass urine. His genitals were completely numb and his feet now felt like he was walking on razor blades. This time the MRI scans showed up numerous brain and spinal lesions, and the diagnosis of MS quickly followed. Three days of intravenous steroids calmed the symptoms, and by the time Craig returned home he was walking, painfully, and urinating often.

The relapse and diagnosis couldn't have come at a worse time for Craig and his wife. Work was stressful and busy, baby Jonah was just three months old, and they were in the middle of renovating their house. Craig managed to keep working, though his vision had not returned to normal yet and he was struggling with a whole host of symptoms. Then, about four months later, he was hit by another relapse. This set the tone for what became an unpleasant pattern over the next four years—a relentless series of relapses, followed by only partial recovery. During this period he was given eighteen doses of steroids and was put on the disease-modifying drugs Betaferon and then Copaxone, which he took for two years before being offered something stronger. 'Everyone at work knew I had MS, there was just no hiding it,' he says. 'I would just do what I could and then go home when I got tired. I was working more in the factory rather than with customers,' he says. 'My family was really supportive through all of this time. My aunties and uncles and grandma and my mum and dad, they really helped me.'

Craig's illness was taking its toll on his relationship though, and when his son Jonah was a year old he and his wife separated. 'We just grew apart. It was a really difficult time for both of us. My symptoms were so extreme. I remember one day Deb brushed against me with her arm and it felt like I'd been hit by a baseball bat,' he recalls. 'And my feet still felt like they were walking on razor blades, so moving around at home was a big effort. I remember taking off my shoes and socks and checking for blood because I couldn't believe there was no actual injury.'

Craig's cognitive function was suffering as well. When Deb used the standard tactic of spelling out words she didn't want Jonah to hear—saying C–A–K–E instead of cake—Craig struggled to understand the words himself. 'Mentally I was going downhill big time,' he says. 'I couldn't do two things at once; I couldn't walk and talk at the same time. It took all my senses just to walk, so if someone came up and talked to me at the same time I'd fall over. Then I'd get cranky with the person who'd come and spoken to me.'

In the end Craig parted from both his marriage and his job, moving into a one-bedroom ground-floor apartment that his uncle helped him buy. Here he was able to share the care of Jonah, whom he looked after for four or five days every fortnight. After a few months he also started working part time as a porter at the local hospital, as part of a rehabilitation scheme to get him back into the workforce. This type of work suited him for a number of reasons. Firstly because the trolleys for patients that he was pushing gave him something to lean on when his legs threatened to give way, and secondly because toilets were everywhere inside the hospital, meaning his frequent need to urinate could be accommodated quite easily. The work suited Craig in another important way: it matched his caring nature and his empathy with the people he was helping. When his health was good he was an excellent addition to the team of friendly hospital staff. When MS delivered him another blow, he disappeared from the wards and corridors for a while and spent time at home recovering.

By 2005 his life was manageable, though he was planning for major disability. 'I bought my apartment based around the fact that I could get a wheelchair in when I was going to need it,' he recalls. 'I've always had a positive attitude, but I started to plan for relapses. I'd be thinking about holidays and I'd say no, I won't go away that month because I'll probably have another relapse.'

Then early in 2006 he was hit with a big one. 'I went blind in my left eye,' he says. 'I took steroids for that, and just as it was getting better I went blind in my right eye as well,' he remembers. Craig was still recovering from his loss of vision when he started experiencing some very disturbing symptoms in his hands. 'My fingers felt like they were two or three inches thick and I couldn't use them properly. I couldn't even open the front door and I had to stop driving.' With these relapses all occurring in the space of three months, Craig's neurologist recommended the chemotherapy drug mitoxantrone in an effort to halt the relapses and buy his body a bit of time. Seen as a last-resort measure in very aggressive forms of MS, chemotherapy is thought to stop relapses completely—but only for a couple of years at most. Given the shocking relapse rate and rapid decline in his health, Craig agreed to give chemo a try. 'I really thought I was screwed,' he says simply. 'I thought in another few months I wouldn't be able to look after my son anymore, the MS was just so bad at that time,' he says. 'I just planned to do everything I wanted to do in the next two or three years, expecting it was going to get ugly after that.'

Craig had yet another dose of steroids and then started chemotherapy. Physically he was well enough to return to his part-time job as a hospital porter, but emotionally he was a wreck. Standing in the hospital lobby waiting to take a break one day he ran into his friend Janine, a midwife he'd met while working on the wards. Janine took one look at Craig and told him frankly, 'You look awful!' and the whole story of his recent relapses, chemotherapy and fears for the future came out. And in that moment, just when his life seemed completely doomed, was the spark of something new. It was a spark that led not only to a wonderful relationship resulting in marriage, but also to the beginning of his recovery.

Most couples can remember where they met. Craig and Janine Wheeler first met one afternoon at the end of a long shift on the maternity ward. Janine was attending the last of three caesareans and unexpectedly the baby had been born seriously ill. 'It was an absolute emergency as far as resuscitation goes and there were lots of doctors and nurses in there helping at the time,' Janine remembers. 'The baby was taken to intensive care and the mother was really worried. I knew she had to spend time with her baby before he was transferred to Melbourne, but everyone was too busy to help me organise it.'

As the minutes ticked by Janine started to get desperate. Then suddenly someone popped up right in front of her and said, 'I'll do it, this lady needs to be with her baby.' That was Craig. Together he and Janine pushed the trolley down to intensive care, moving beds and other furniture so that mum and baby could share a few precious moments of closeness. 'We stood there watching this lady talk to her baby and watching her world unfold. We felt good that we had made a difference,' Janine says. 'I think a bond formed between us that day that never went away.'

In the following weeks Craig and Janine occasionally saw each other on the wards, and slowly they became friends. It was several months before Craig shared the fact that he had MS. 'I was floored,' Janine says. 'I had only ever seen him when he was well. Whenever he had a relapse he stayed off work, so I had no concept he was unwell—I just saw him as a funny, caring, delightful guy.'

When Janine met Craig in the lobby that July morning after he'd started chemotherapy, she knew straight away that something was badly amiss. 'He just looked broken, and I thought that was so wrong. He deserved to be well and happy, to receive some of the care that he gave to other people.'

Janine was already aware of the work of The Gawler Foundation and the MS retreats that were held there. When she got home that day she printed off some information and later phoned Craig to tell him what she'd found out. It may seem like a strange path to romance, but a week later they became a couple. They also booked their first 'holiday' together: a week in the Yarra Valley Living Centre attending George Jelinek and Ian Gawler's Taking Control of MS retreat.

In the three months leading up to the retreat, Janine accompanied Craig when he went for his chemotherapy injections. She quizzed the staff about the treatment and its chances of success. 'I remember talking to the nurse who was giving the chemo and I asked how many people were doing it, and he said twenty. So I asked him how many of them were improving and he said none. Then I asked him how many were getting worse and he said that most were staying the same,' Janine recalls. 'That was about the best we could hope for.'

Janine also watched as Craig filled up on schnitzel burgers and chips after the treatments, knowing that he'd be too nauseous to eat much by the following day. 'His diet was really dreadful,' Janine laughs. 'He even took me to a fast-food place during one of our first dates.' Craig agrees, citing his busy trade background as the reason for his reliance on pies, chips, chocolates and burgers—the staples of a junk-food diet. 'In my twenties I had this busy lifestyle where I got used to grabbing something to eat when I could. And it was usually junk,' he says. 'I wasn't overweight though, I just ate badly.'

The night before leaving for the retreat in October 2006, Craig and Janine had one last meal of steak and chips. Craig was still unsure whether the week was a good idea. 'When Janine first mentioned the retreat to me I had heard of it before, but I just thought it was hippy stuff,' he says. 'But I was really out of options and I was open-minded at the start that this could work. Still, I was pretty worried about the food,' he admits. On the four-hour drive to the retreat, Craig stopped off at a bakery and bought cheese and ham croissants. He was clinging to his old habits for as long as he possibly could.

Walking into the peaceful haven of the Yarra Valley, this was all about to change. Craig looked at the plates of food that were placed in front of him and came out with a whole range of expletives. 'I was pretty rude,' he says, 'but some days I just couldn't believe what they were making me eat.' Janine took the wholefood, plant-based diet more in her stride. For her, meditation was the biggest problem. 'As soon as we went into the meditation sanctuary I just started giggling,' she says. 'In the end it got that I couldn't go in there at all. I knew it was important for everyone's healing and I didn't want to spoil it for them,' she says. Craig, however, took to meditation straight away, finding it a profound and nurturing experience right from the start.

'Once before I'd had a massage and at the end the guy had asked if I wanted to have my energy centred,' remembers Craig. 'I said yes, and it was the lightest touch massage I'd ever had. But he warned me that afterwards I might get a bit upset.' Sure enough, that evening Craig had started crying every time he closed his eyes. Being introduced to meditation at the retreat reminded him of that experience—of the way the mind and body are linked. Craig now describes meditation as relaxation for the brain. 'I don't know the answers to meditation but I do enjoy it,' he says. 'If you're only working on the physical side of things then you're not really getting the whole picture. Once you start to get into the stillness, that's where the healing happens.'

Halfway through the week, things began to jell for both Craig and Janine. With pages of notes to explain the scientific rationale behind the diet, they took themselves off to the nearest supermarket to stock up on extra supplies. 'We didn't consider it sneaking out,' says Craig. 'We were using the knowledge we'd been given and taking control of our health. It was all good food that we bought—fruit, vegetables, nuts, seeds.'

The retreat also started an emotional growth in both of them, and allowed Janine to confront some of her own issues. 'The week was not just about MS, it was also about forgiveness and about managing stress,' she says. 'It was also a big reality check for me. There were people there at every stage of disability and I remember looking around thinking that we could be in a bit of strife with Craig's health if this doesn't work out. Perhaps before that I'd been in the first glow of a new relationship, but once I got to the retreat it was time to confront MS.'

By the end of the week Craig was convinced by the major aspects of the recovery program—diet, vitamin D, exercise and meditation. Driving back home he and Janine noticed the bustle of life creeping back in, the traffic on the roads, the noises of city life. They also noticed the smells from the fast-food outlets, and for a little while Craig was still a bit tempted. 'I could smell the burgers from the car while we were waiting at the traffic lights, and I thought ooh, that smells good,' remembers Craig. 'But Janine looked at me and said "smells like wheelchairs" and that was that.'

Janine had already noticed an improvement in Craig's energy levels while they were at the retreat, and this continued once they got home. He still needed a two-hour sleep most afternoons to get him through the day, but he was generally more lively and optimistic. He had his vitamin D levels checked and they were below the recommended amount, so he started supplementing. And he completely transformed his diet, embracing the new regime with a vigour that surprised everyone. 'I think he applied the same kind of mental attitude to his recovery diet that he'd used in training for marathons in the past,' Janine explains. Craig started juicing vegetables daily, and in time he even started growing his own. 'I was a real beginner gardener,' he says, 'so to start with I'd plant things far too close together, but I soon learned. And I found with the food that you have to put a bit of effort in and then it tastes magnificent.'

Within weeks, the exact same meals he'd been so rude about at the retreat became firm favourites. 'I came to really love carrot cake and spinach and all the Asian greens,' he laughs. 'Now I wouldn't eat any other way.'

Knowing that it could take five years to stabilise using diet and lifestyle, Craig continued with the chemotherapy injections, though now he turned up to his appointments with pieces of fruit in his hands. 'He found the chemo a lot easier to handle without all that junk food on board,' says Janine. 'He bounced back much quicker and didn't get so sick.'

In January 2007 Craig and Janine moved in together, into a two-storey house. 'Some of my friends were concerned, asking how Craig was going to manage to get up the stairs!' says Janine incredulously. 'I told them he's going to walk, which is exactly what happened.'

To begin with Craig's recovery was marked by a lack of relapses. He was still struggling with symptoms—bladder and bowel issues, restless legs and feet, numbness and cognitive problems. But at least there was no new damage to add to the physical burden.

As time went on, however, and the relapses stayed away, some of these symptoms started to recede. 'I reckon it got to the point where I was urinating twelve times a night. Gradually that got less and less,' Craig says, noting that he no longer needed to take a bottle with him on car journeys in case he got caught out.

The retreat was the first of many trips and holidays for Craig and Janine, though none were quite as intense as that first one. 'It was really important for us to always have something to look forward to, and we made a point of recording our holidays in photo albums so we could look back and remember them,' says Janine. 'There was always something planned, even if it was just a weekend away with the kids.'

They decided to both continue to work part time, believing that a healthy and balanced lifestyle would be achieved more easily with that arrangement. Janine's three children from a previous marriage and Craig's son all spent large amounts of time with them at the house. When the kids were there, Craig and

Janine concentrated on family life; when it was just the two of them, they spent more time working. 'If we both worked full time I think we'd struggle to maintain the lifestyle,' says Janine. 'It's amazing how we get by on part-time wages. We'll never be loaded, but we're rich in other ways.'

In April 2008 that richness grew to include marriage. 'We'd been talking about getting married ever since we'd been together,' Craig says. 'It really was an instant connection between us, a real meeting of souls.'

When it came to finding a suitable venue, Janine felt The Gawler Foundation was an obvious choice, with George Jelinek and Ian Gawler acting as witnesses. 'It was the place where hope began,' she says simply.

On the day of the wedding, gale-force winds meant that the actual ceremony had to be held indoors. 'Ian told us that windy weather is a very good omen for marriages according to Tibetan monks,' says Craig. 'So we were quite happy with that.'

After a simple ceremony the couple had lunch in the Yarra Valley with current MS retreat participants, before returning home to Geelong.

Everything stayed on track with Craig's health. He stopped needing to sleep in the afternoons, his walking became stronger, his feet were less restless at night, and his mental alertness kept improving.

Still working at the hospital as a porter, he was offered the chance to train as a theatre technician, and he took it. 'I had to do three months of training and six months of study for that,' says Craig. His mind and body were ready for the challenge, and a short while later he trained as a plaster technician as well, learning to attend to all the people with broken arms, wrists, ankles and legs who presented at the hospital. 'That was another six weeks of specialist training and a year of study,' he adds.

Then, in the winter of 2010, four years after his last relapse, Craig felt numbness and weakness in his right arm. 'My arm just stopped moving—it felt like it had no power in it,' he says. Craig went back to his neurologist, who prescribed the usual steroid treatment. Craig also asked to have his vitamin D level checked, and was astounded to find it had dropped to just 60 nmol/L, way below the recommended minimum. 'That was a real kick in the bum for me. I just hadn't been taking my supplements because I'd put the bottle away in the pantry instead of leaving it out in the kitchen,' says Craig. 'That relapse was a real blow, but when I realised how low my vitamin D was I felt I had a good explanation for it.'

Craig took a megadose of vitamin D to boost his levels, and continued his recovery through diet, meditation and exercise. He also decided to briefly take Copaxone again. With her medical background Janine was able to give Craig the injections, so that part was easier than before. But psychologically, taking medication again proved very difficult for Craig, who had always disliked drugs of any kind. 'He just had this look of defeat in his eyes when I was giving him the injections,' Janine recalls. 'Like when you put a dog into a bath and they look at you as if to say "Oh God, why are you doing this to me"?' she says. After only a few days Craig decided to stop the drugs. 'When I took them it made me feel like a patient again, so I reckoned I was better off without them,' he says. Since then, his symptoms have continued to improve, with no further relapses.

By 2011 Craig was walking further and more easily than he had been for years, but running still seemed off-limits. Thinking back to his marathon-running days, Craig had tested his body a few times to see whether he could remember what to do. For a long time he couldn't. The breakthrough finally came early in 2012 when he was giving one of the kids some batting practice at cricket. 'I'd gone in to bowl and I found that I just couldn't get the action right if I was only walking,' he remembers. 'So I decided to have a go at running. I'd tried a few times over the years and my body just hadn't responded, but this time it worked,' he says happily. After this success Craig decided to join the kids when they were running laps of the oval in training for cross-country races at school. 'I just have to work at it a little bit and teach my muscles what to do again. It'll be worth it because I really love running as an activity.'

Back in July 2006 Craig Wheeler thought his life was over. Today both he and Janine see their lives as happy, healthy and fulfilled. 'We love our caring roles at work and I think we've got a very exciting future ahead of us,' Janine says. 'When I look at Craig I don't see illness and disability. In the six years we've been together, every year he's been healthier than the one before,' she says.

Craig is quick to agree. 'Life's going really well and my health is going really well. That has been the big goal: I think if my health is going well then everything else just flows from that.'

As for the future, Craig expects to be able to achieve pretty much whatever he wants. 'I have a very positive outlook about where I'm going,' he says. 'Janine and the kids are a big part in that. Back in 2006 I wasn't sure I could bring another person into my life because my health was such a mess. But it's definitely not all doom and gloom anymore,' he says. 'I think now that if I wanted to, I could go back to work full time; things are just getting better and better.'

5

CONVERSION OF A TRUE SCEPTIC

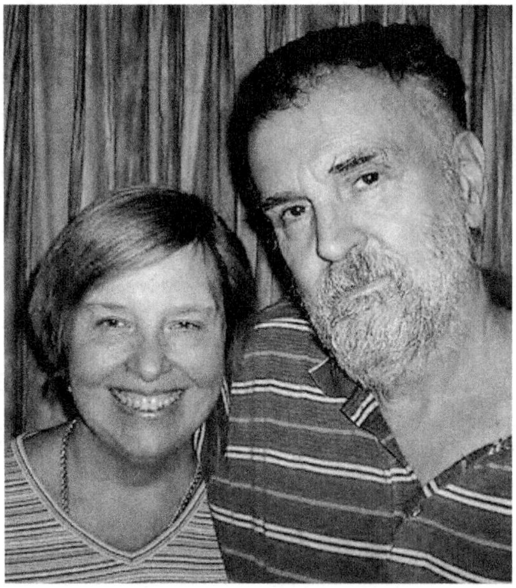

GINNY BILLSON

Ginny Billson is rather good at puzzles. Magic tricks fascinate her, and her favourite books are detective stories. As she turns the pages and watches the many plots unfold, she isn't only focusing on the characters, but also the psychology of what makes people behave the way they do. She is looking for evidence. Once she has all the facts, her analytical mind takes over, methodically working through the data to come up with a solution. It is usually correct.

Ginny was born in Melbourne, Australia, in 1949, the only child of Lithuanian migrant parents. As a girl she used to drive everyone mad with her questioning, her constant need to know 'why?' Of course, many five-year-olds go through that stage; Ginny reached it earlier than most, and she never grew out of it. She questioned her mum as she got ready for work in the mornings. She questioned her opera-singing grandma, who lived with them in their small suburban house. She couldn't question her dad, because he'd left soon after Ginny was born. And she soon learned not to question her stepdad, a veteran of the Second World War who had problems with drinking and gambling.

There wasn't much money around while Ginny was growing up. Her mum worked hard to establish the family, taking a job as a kitchen scrubber at the Mercy Hospital to survive financially. Her good language skills and ability to speak English meant that she soon moved on to other things, working in real estate for a while before accepting a secretarial position at a Melbourne hospital. 'She worked really hard and by the end of her career she had elevated herself to the head of secretarial support in radiology,' Ginny says. 'She was, and still is, very intelligent.'

Like mother, like daughter. Ginny inherited her mum's sharp thinking and attention to detail. She was good at schoolwork, though it took a while for her true talents to be recognised. 'I was actually quite a terror when I went to primary school because I got very bored,' remembers Ginny. 'I was always chatting, being disruptive, and there were a couple of teachers who told me I would never amount to anything.' That comment cut deep, right to the heart of the migrant's sensitivity about making it in the new country. 'They were really quite cruel, and I quietly set out to change their opinion,' says Ginny.

When she reached high school things improved markedly. Now there were greater academic challenges, more interesting problems for her to focus on. Home life wasn't great, but Ginny blocked out the worst of it by burying herself in books. She enjoyed many of the regular teenage activities too—swimming, horseriding, friends. But it was books that held the greatest joy, with detective stories topping the list. 'I loved reading and I was forever pestering Mum to take me to the library because of course we couldn't afford to buy many books ourselves,' she says. 'I loved whodunit stories, but I enjoyed science fiction as well. I was fascinated by the theories those stories were based on; they opened up a whole new frontier for me.'

When Ginny was fourteen she got a Saturday job at a local department store. This was mainly to contribute to the family income, but she also really enjoyed it. 'I started off in the knitwear and children's toy section. They actually told me I had a great future at the store, but I decided that wasn't what I wanted to do for the rest of my life,' she says. After a couple of years Ginny moved on to waitressing, and later became assistant chef at a nearby reception centre. By that time her grandma had passed away. She and her mum escaped from a rather tough situation at home and set up together, Ginny continuing to pay her way with part-time jobs while she finished high school.

Then, due to her exceptional grades, she was awarded a scholarship to study science at the University of Melbourne. She started the degree course, but by the end of the first year she found she was getting rather bored. Thinking medicine might be more interesting she applied for a transfer, and luckily her scholarship was transferred too. That was essential: by the end of second year Ginny was working as a lab technician at the local hospital as well as continuing with her assistant chef duties to make ends meet. The busy lifestyle suited her, and she thrived on the study too. 'Medicine was great fun. I found it a challenge and I really enjoyed it.'

A couple of years into her medical degree she met her future husband, Alex. 'He hung around for a while, then he hung around for a bit longer, and he's still hanging around now,' she says gratefully. Alex, a senior lab engineer at La Trobe University, was a few years older than Ginny. 'It was good to have someone around who was non-medical, someone sane,' she laughs. They were married by the time she had graduated.

There was neither time nor money for a honey-moon at that point in their lives. Ginny completed residencies at various local hospitals to develop her skills and discover which area of medicine she wanted to specialise in. Her questioning mind influenced the decision. 'At that stage it was really a toss-up between pathology and paediatrics,' she remembers. 'I was drawn to pathology because it's a bit like detective work. I like to suss out what's going on, what the motivation is behind things. I loved pathology because you use lots of pieces of information to arrive at an answer,' she explains.

So Ginny embarked on the five-year training program in pathology. Two years into the course, she and Alex were finally able to go on an extended honeymoon. 'I had a year off from working and studying and we travelled overseas for about six months, staying in hostels and visiting lots of wonderful places,' Ginny recalls. By the time they returned, Ginny was pregnant. 'A souvenir from Paris, or perhaps the Leningrad Express,' she smiles. Back in Melbourne their son Lawrence was born; after the birth Ginny returned to her pathology post part time until Lawrence was old enough to start school. 'I decided I had worked out what caused these things called babies, so we only had the one child,' she quips. 'I'm a quick learner.'

Life was busy with a preschooler and a full-time job, but Alex was hugely supportive. As Lawrence grew from toddler to teenager, Ginny's pathology work blossomed into a highly successful and fulfilling career. If she'd still cared about the cruel remarks of her primary school teachers, she could have disproved them many times over.

By 1995 Ginny had spent thousands of hours peering into microscopes, analysing tissue samples to diagnose disease or determine causes of death. Her articles and research papers had been published in numerous pathology journals and she was a well-respected member of the medical community. Working 80 or 90 hours a week was not uncommon, and to top it off she'd recently decided to study business management. 'After that I was appointed head of the department, which was also great fun to begin with,' she says. However, a change in government brought widespread privatisation within the public hospital system where Ginny was working. It was an unsettling time for all medical staff, and Ginny was now responsible for a large team. 'There was a lot of cost-cutting that came with corporatisation, and a huge chance of people being made redundant,' she says. 'As head of department that was quite stressful; I was right in the thick of it and I was definitely not enjoying it.'

With a very volatile work situation to contend with, Ginny really needed her home life to keep running smoothly. It didn't. At exactly that moment her son Lawrence, who had just turned seventeen, announced that he was running off to live in San Francisco. It appeared to be a rather wild and badly thought-out plan, and there was a girl involved. 'It all sounded perfectly okay to him, but it didn't sound so good to us,' muses Ginny.

She dropped everything to respond to the family crisis. 'Alex and I realised we couldn't stop him going, if he was really determined. But we came up with a plan to turn it into a mother–son bonding experience, to find out what was going on, meet this girl and see if things were really going to work out,' she says. Lawrence agreed. As an incentive, Ginny booked a two-week tour to Mexico afterwards, which Lawrence could only enjoy if he chose to leave San Francisco with her. 'It was obviously very stressful and I was thinking crikey, is he actually going to stay there?' To Ginny's enormous relief, he didn't. 'Within a week he could see this wasn't what he wanted, and we started to look forward to spending the rest of the trip together,' she says.

It was just before Christmas 1995 when Ginny and Lawrence boarded the bus in Los Angeles at the start of their fifteen-day guided tour down the west coast. The first few days passed smoothly enough, through San Diego then across the Mexican border into Tijuana. On Christmas Eve they stopped in the coastal city of Ensenada. Still recovering from the many stresses of the past month, and in keeping with the festive season, Ginny enjoyed a few margaritas that night. The next day she woke up with a bit of a headache and double vision. The headache was understandable, but the double vision was more of a mystery. Of course, her questioning mind wondered what had caused it, and the margaritas from the night before were high on the list of suspects for the first few hours. But when the headache wore off and the double vision worsened, Ginny used her medical knowledge to widen the search. By evening she was seriously panicking.

'Double vision is not a good symptom. I could think of 150 things that might cause it, and all 150 of them were ghastly,' she admits. Interestingly enough, multiple sclerosis didn't feature on the list at all. 'There I was, on a bus in the wilds of Mexico, and I was sure that the rare brain infection or rapidly lethal tumour was going to end my trip sooner rather than later,' she admits.

The tour guide was helpful and kind, arranging for Ginny to visit an emergency department on their next day's stopover in Phoenix, Arizona. For the second time that trip, Ginny was hugely relieved that Lawrence had decided to stay with her. 'He was growing up fast and was a great comfort to me,' she says. When a CAT scan and neurological review showed there was no serious lesion, doctors diagnosed sixth nerve palsy, a common and benign condition. 'They said I should resume my trip, relax and it would pass,' says Ginny.

Mother and son rejoined the tour in Las Vegas and continued on through Yosemite, San Francisco and back to Los Angeles via Disneyland and Universal Studios. 'By that time the double vision was lessening and I was able to start enjoying the tourist experience,' remembers Ginny. 'We flew home from LA and by the time we landed everything was normal again.'

Back in Australia she consulted a trusted neurologist, and he confirmed that sixth nerve palsies were quite common and usually needed no further management. 'I was very reassured, and I forgot about the evil experience and just enjoyed the memories of an eventful trip,' she says.

Two problems seemed to have been resolved over that month, but Ginny was still left with a third: the situation at work. With a tense political atmosphere and the threat of mass redundancy hanging over everyone's head, her pathology job went through a very unsettled period for more than a year. Then, just before Ginny's 48th birthday, the whole department was made redundant.

'That's when I developed some more strange symptoms,' Ginny remembers. 'I lost the taste in half my mouth, and I was very unstable on one side when I was walking. My left leg just gave way, though I didn't actually fall over.' One morning Ginny sat down and found that one half of her buttocks felt really cold, and the other half felt numb. 'I thought uh oh, that's not right, obviously the brain tumour is growing,' she says, all too aware of how these symptoms played with her normally logical mind.

She was admitted to hospital and underwent a battery of tests, including MRIs and a lumbar puncture. Within a couple of days she received the MS diagnosis.

'It was the most horrendous news and I was devastated,' she says. Steroids eased the symptoms, but nothing eased the fear. 'It was already a traumatic time at work, not knowing what was to follow the redundancy. MS came on top of that and it was very hard to cope with. Being in the medical world you hear about the worst side of every disease—all the terrible situations that can happen.'

Ginny decided to become an expert on MS, reading every medical textbook and research paper she could lay her hands on. 'And then I ignored it,' she says honestly.

Unfortunately, MS didn't ignore her. She was hit with repeated relapses, around three each year. Despite this Ginny managed to secure, and retain, a part-time pathology job. 'It was at a different hospital with a small pathology unit and I really enjoyed it. And it was great not to be working 70 hours a week anymore,' she recalls. In fact, it was vital. Some of Ginny's relapses were unsettling and annoying; others were downright frightening, and two put her in hospital. 'I had one episode where my balance was severely affected, and I couldn't really walk,' she remembers. 'That was a bad one and I needed intensive rehabilitation afterwards.' Another episode started with mild dizziness and progressed to feeling like the very worst type of sea-sickness. 'Every time I lifted my head off the pillow I vomited. I needed an ambulance to take me to hospital because I couldn't get vertical,' she remembers bleakly.

In between her two major relapses she experienced a range of milder attacks of numbness and double vision that were still quite worrying and disabling.

But it was the hospital stays that affected her most, requiring high-dose steroids that left her feeling very tired and gloomy. 'I was getting quite depressed after a couple of years because it was all so horrendous,' she admits. 'Every time I had an episode I felt like I'd been hit over the head because of the enormous fatigue that set in. I was also taking interferon, which made me feel pretty awful and didn't seem to be having much effect on the relapses,' she says.

Life was manageable, but often very difficult. 'I really couldn't see an end to it, and from time to time the concept of suicide did come into the piece,' she says bluntly. Ginny admits that for the first time in her life she could understand why people might decide to end it all. 'That was mainly when I was most fatigued after the high-dose cortisones and the hospitalisations,' she says. 'They were scary episodes, uncomfortable and fatiguing, and I just wanted to give up, basically.' For about a week afterwards she remembers thinking, 'Gee, if that's all I've got to look forward to then I'm over it.' Luckily, once her symptoms settled and the cortisone wore off she bounced back a little. 'Those depressing thoughts would wane and I would start to feel a bit better,' she recalls.

It had only taken a few short years, but Ginny's life had changed dramatically since the onset of MS.

After decades of successfully juggling a career, family, research, committee work and social engagements, her orderly world was crumbling with the disruption of continual relapses that left her feeling hopeless and desperate. 'It was certainly scary, knowing that I was on medication and possibly this was the best I was ever going to be,' she says. Then, over the New Year of 2001, Ginny attended an MS peer support workers Christmas gathering.

'I got talking to someone there and they told me about a book that I ought to read called *Taking Control of Multiple Sclerosis,'* she remembers. Being sceptical by nature, she was immediately on high alert, looking out for false claims and bad science. And Ginny was no ordinary sceptic: she was actually a paid-up member of the Sceptics Society, a dedicated seeker of truth in all matters. 'A lot of the Sceptics Society activities are aimed at debunking theories, particularly ones that take advantage of people emotionally and financially,' she says. 'I like things to be logical and I hate seeing people assuming things that are actually incorrect. That's my detective nature, my need to get to the bottom of things.'

So Ginny took the book and not only read, but also analysed, the research papers on diet, exercise, vitamin D and meditation. She put the theory to the test, and it passed scrutiny. 'I thought there was good evidence behind it and that what George Jelinek was saying made absolute sense, once you understood the underlying science of the whole thing,' she says. 'It is actually profoundly logical for the sceptical mind.'

Some of her medical peers may have had little time for the lifestyle approach, but Ginny was convinced. 'Some of the medical fraternity don't accept the holistic view because it fits a different paradigm,' she explains. 'It's not as simple as 1 plus 1 equals 2. There are a lot of factors involved so it's more like 1 plus 32 equals 33. There are so many different concepts to come up with the final answer, but each input has a logical sequence and a logical outcome.'

Convinced that lifestyle and dietary changes could in theory make a difference to MS, Ginny committed to putting these into practice and applying them to her own life. Right in the midst of her debilitating relapses, and with her spirits still rather low from the constant fatigue and medication, she methodically worked through the recommendations, considering what she needed to change in order to comply. Her diet in 2001 was not great. She was quite significantly overweight, she ate the wrong foods, and she usually ate too much of them. Ginny's was a typical Western diet, full of meat, dairy and some processed food. 'I used to eat a lot of ice cream and cheese, though I was never really into sweets and lollies,' she says. 'After reading the research I decided to follow the Swank recommendations, keeping my saturated fat below 15 grams a day. I never ate meat and I removed all dairy from the household. I really think dairy has a lot of negative aspects so I'm very religious about that.' Ginny's vegetable and fruit intake increased, and her diet became based around plants and seafood. When she found she was missing eggs in her diet, she did some research and decided that well-sourced organic eggs shouldn't be a problem. 'I really missed my eggs, so I do now have one a week,' she says. 'Since 2001 I have eaten really well, but I still eat too much of it,' she concedes. Nevertheless her weight has dropped by 15kg (33lb), and is still gradually going down.

Ginny found the evidence on vitamin D and its role in MS so compelling that she followed the recommendations to the letter. 'I really think that is vital for recovery,' she says.

After twenty years in a sedentary job, with walking the dog her only exercise, Ginny was a long way off her ideal level of fitness. She began very slowly, incorporating just a little bit of swimming and walking into her weekly routine.

Meditation was a new and interesting concept, and one she found her own answer to. 'I really got rather bored with sitting down quietly, but I did like the mindfulness aspect of it. So when I went for a walk I started to concentrate on feeling my feet on the ground.' She did the same while swimming, paying attention to how her body was moving and feeling as she exercised. 'I started doing this type of active meditation two or three times a day,' she recalls. 'Occasionally I would also practise sitting meditation as well.'

In 2002, and again in 2007, Ginny chose to attend an MS retreat to help her incorporate the changes into her everyday life. She likens this to the process of immunisation. 'Reading the evidence and the research was like having a vaccination,' she says. 'Then when I attended the retreats it was like getting a booster shot.'

By the end of 2001 Ginny had incorporated what she felt were the key elements for recovery into her life, and she continued to take interferon. Having set the process in motion, all that remained was to sit back and watch to see what kind of results might follow. Of course, Ginny was only interested in 'real' results—tangible evidence that the course of MS was being positively affected by the changes she had made. What happened next was very heartening. With the disease so active just prior to making her lifestyle changes, it would have been too much to hope for an immediate halt to the relapses. And, indeed, that is not what happened. But within six months the intensity of the relapses, and the time between them, subtly improved. This gave Ginny hope that the regime was working, and that the theory she had put her faith in was sound. Nevertheless, she had some very frightening episodes to live through before she felt the disease had been stabilised.

Her first relapse after making the diet and lifestyle changes was a peculiar bout of jaw pain. Fearing her teeth were falling apart, Ginny went to the dentist, only to discover that it was an MS-related symptom.

'It was really strange and very unsettling,' she says. 'Every minute and a half I'd get this stabbing pain in one of my back teeth. It was so regular I could set my watch to it.'

Six months later she developed a patch of intense itchiness over her left shoulder blade. 'It drove me absolutely nuts for a while, but it turned out to be a fading symptom, getting less severe over a period of a week,' she remembers.

Another six months passed without incident and Ginny was starting to relax and enjoy life a bit more. Around this time she also found that her overall level of physical and mental wellbeing was improving. 'As I started to recover, my episodes weren't so fatiguing—it was more mild and general,' she remembers. 'Whereas before, during a relapse, the terrible fatigue would hit me and really pull me down.'

Her next relapse was actually one of the most terrifying Ginny had ever experienced, although she didn't end up in hospital and the symptoms cleared up quite quickly. Again it was episodic in nature, but this time affecting the functioning of her whole body. 'I'd be sitting down talking to someone and every minute and a half my mouth and brain just stopped working,' she recalls. Around ten seconds later, normal functioning resumed. Then, regular as clockwork, the same thing would happen, repeatedly throughout the day. 'If I was walking my legs just stopped; if I was talking my mouth just stopped. It was the weirdest thing and quite terrifying in its own way,' she says.

'I went to my neurologist and he had a long name for it, which reassured me a bit.' He also prescribed Tegretol, which helped to clear it up, and within a few weeks the symptoms had tapered off and disappeared.

The next eighteen months of Ginny's life were peppered with occasional mild relapses—numbness and double vision, then spasms in her hands, as if someone was squeezing her thumbs. The final relapse was marked by slight dizziness and a feeling of being a little unsteady on her feet. Of course, Ginny didn't know it was the final relapse at the time. But ten years later she can look back with relief and know that seven years of MS attacks ended right there. For good.

With the relapses under control, Ginny continued building on her level of fitness. In 2007 she started working with a personal trainer at her local gym. As soon as she began building up her muscle strength, she found that her residual fatigue disappeared. 'I still had some mild, general fatigue at that time, even though I hadn't had a relapse for around five years. But after the gym work that has never been an issue for me again.'

For a while the fitness protocol was a tough one for Ginny to adhere to, and she says she really had to take herself in hand. 'For those first few years I was hugely overweight,' she admits. 'I was very unfit and not really able to do much at all, and I couldn't run to save myself.'

But as the weight dropped off, the relapses tapered off and the fatigue lifted, Ginny watched her fitness improve. 'Over the last ten years I have definitely got a lot more active, and I feel so much better for it,' she says happily.

Now aged 63, her current weekly schedule begins with a 45-minute intensive workout with Mila, her personal trainer. 'I've been working with her for four years and we've become good friends,' she says. Then every Saturday morning Ginny lines up with a group of other ladies for boot camp. 'It's a bit less intense than my private training. We trot or struggle round the football oval and do weights for about an hour.' In addition, Ginny visits the gym once or twice more during the week, running on the treadmill and lifting weights to improve her strength. 'I've found it really helps with my balance as well.'

It's a wonder she has time for so much exercise, because Ginny's life is once again extraordinarily full. She sings with a local ladies choir, is a very active member of Rotary, and talks to groups about her MS story. 'I like to do things that are good for me and good for the community, and have fun while I'm doing it,' she says simply.

Most importantly, Ginny is still working for three days a week at the Royal Women's Hospital in Melbourne. 'I'm a senior sessional histopathologist. I still do diagnostic work, which I love, and perinatal work on stillborn babies, and a bit of teaching,' she says.

'And in my spare time I write research papers,' she laughs.

She has no plans for retirement. Indeed, in such specialised areas of medicine it is common for doctors to keep working well into their seventies. 'There are people in my department at the moment who are around that age. If I'm still up to it, and I certainly expect to be, then I would like to do the same.'

Her husband Alex, the sane one, has had the good sense to retire. He now spends part of his time restoring old cars, including a 1930s Model A Ford that he was hoping to have ready for their son Lawrence's wedding. So that story has a happy ending too.

Looking back on her whole experience with MS, Ginny is relieved to be able to put some distance between herself and the horror of those first few years after diagnosis. As a result, in her analytical way, she now views it as interesting and curious, as much as she once saw it as terrifying and depressing. She doesn't claim to have been cured of the disease, but knows she has kept MS at bay with the diet and lifestyle changes she implemented back in 2001. Her recovery is incredible, but it is no mystery.

And that, to someone as sceptical as Ginny Billson, is extremely satisfying.

6

PROVING THEM WRONG

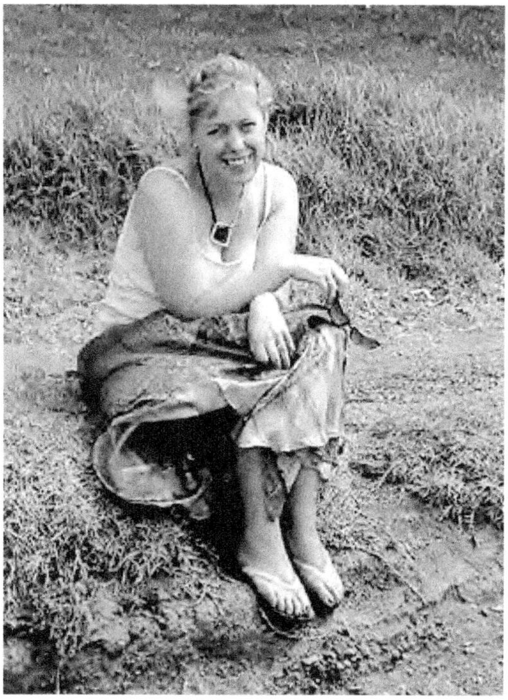

CARRIE PHILLISKIRK

Whenever people try to put limitations on Carrie Philliskirk's life, she tends to come out fighting. It's a gentle fight, but it's one she almost always wins. When Carrie was 21, for example, her father predicted she'd never make it through the tough training course to become a nurse in the British Royal Navy. She was determined to prove him wrong.

'I'd just spent three years at nursing college and when I finished there were no hospital jobs at all,' she says. However, the Gulf War meant that at least the armed forces were recruiting nurses. Carrie decided to apply to the Royal Navy, which involved seven weeks of rigorous military training. 'Dad said I'd never be able to stand the discipline,' she remembers. 'It was physically quite a challenge. I wasn't unfit, but I certainly wasn't prepared for the demands of the course,' Carrie admits. 'It had nothing to do with nursing. I had to learn how to fire a gun and maintain it, complete assault courses and spend days with a backpack tramping through the countryside.' Carrie survived the course, and was successfully deployed to the Royal Naval Hospital in Gosport, Hampshire. 'It felt really good to prove Dad wrong,' she laughs, still with a ring of satisfaction in her voice after twenty years.

Carrie grew up in Sunderland in the north-east of England. The city is known for its industrial landscape and areas of deprivation, but Carrie's memory of it is very different. 'We lived in a lovely place. My parents were middle-class professionals, and they both worked, so I had quite a nice upbringing,' she remembers. 'And the people of Sunderland were always so friendly, chatting to you in the streets,' she says.

Carrie was an only child, but would rather not have been. 'I didn't have an unhappy childhood but I always felt under pressure,' she recalls. 'My mum especially had very high expectations of me, of what I should do, and I always felt like a little bit of an under-achiever.'

The stress of never quite getting the results that were expected followed Carrie throughout her school years. Starting off as quiet and introverted, she opened up as a teenager, finding a large social group and becoming more rebellious. 'I could have been academic like my parents wanted, but I was far too busy,' she says. 'I was really musical and I played guitar and trumpet and I spent my teens going from band to band.' At school she tended to do adequately, but never rose to the top of the class. For high school Carrie felt she was 'shipped off' to an all-girls Catholic school, though she was not Catholic. 'It was seen to be better educationally, and the expectation was that I would get higher grades,' she says. 'It didn't work out that way.'

In fact, when the time came for her final exams, Carrie failed abysmally. This left her rather stuck. She had been planning to study social work, 'though Lord knows why', she admits. Another option was the police force, but they were not recruiting at the time. 'Yet again I felt like I was a huge disappointment to my parents and family.'

Then Carrie found a course that didn't need too many qualifications, and she fell into nursing. Somewhat to her surprise, she discovered that she not only loved it but she was also very good at it. 'I really enjoyed it and I loved being around people and having the opportunity to care for them in whatever situation they found themselves—to make a difference,' she says.

Joining the Royal Navy seemed like the only way to gain employment at the end of her studies. Carrie's determination to get through the military training was not just driven by her father's doubts, but by her desire to start working as a nurse. 'I'd finally found something that I was really good at,' she recalls. 'I really felt drawn to it and I couldn't wait to get started.'

Carrie travelled to the south of England to start her nursing career. It was shift work, of course, and it was in the emergency department that Carrie worked very happily for the first few years. The social life was good too, and in 1994 she met her future husband Ian at a party. He was working as an electrical technician in the Navy, and it turned out that he had also grown up in Sunderland, just two streets away from Carrie's childhood home. 'That was the ice-breaker—the fact that we'd gone to the other end of the country in order to meet each other,' she says. From that moment their relationship blossomed.

Four years later their first child, Emily, was born. By that time Carrie was working as a tri-service instructor at Aldershot. There were very few women in that position so she was a bit of a novelty. Becoming pregnant increased the novelty value, and her bosses in the Navy weren't sure how to approach her. 'They ignored me,' laughs Carrie. 'I had a year off and then briefly went back to Gosport. But Ian and I couldn't both be in the Navy and have children, so in the end I left.'

Adapting to life with a new baby was tiring, especially as Ian was often deployed and could be away for months at a time. 'I just had to get on and manage,' Carrie says. 'I found that I got very tired, but I thought it was just the demands of work and motherhood.'

Then, when Emily was four months old, some strange things started happening to Carrie's hands. 'I was hanging out the washing on the line, and every time I went to put a peg on with my right hand I dropped it,' Carrie remembers. 'I just did this repeatedly and I thought it was odd, but again I put it down to being a new mum and perhaps the hormones.' It was the same when Carrie made a cup of coffee. First she spilt the coffee, then she spilt the water, and finally she spilt the milk. 'I had always been very clumsy as a child—my grandad used to call me a bull in a china shop. So I found excuses for what was happening and it almost became a joke,' she says.

Carrie was still breastfeeding Emily at that time, but a month later she stopped. That's when she noticed a problem with the vision in her right eye. 'The colours weren't as vivid and it became very painful at the back of my eye and quite blurred.' Carrie went to an optician, where she was tested and referred to a specialist. 'He diagnosed optic neuritis, but said it was nothing to worry about. I remember asking whether it could be multiple sclerosis, but the ophthalmologist said no, that I was far too well for that to be a possibility,' she says.

After two months Carrie's vision returned to normal, though she was still dropping things and feeling extremely tired. 'Life just carried on. These symptoms bothered me a bit, but they didn't stop me from doing anything.'

Two years later, as Carrie and Ian were busy organising their overseas wedding, the optic neuritis reappeared in her other eye. 'I think it was stress related,' says Carrie. 'I was trying to plan our wedding in Mexico and arrange childcare for Emily. It was similar to the previous time—I couldn't pick out colours and I had pain at the back of my eye,' she recalls. Again it lasted for a few weeks before settling down.

By this time Carrie was working again, in the emergency department of the local town hospital. She and Ian had a second baby, Adam, and then decided to move back up to Sunderland. 'Ian left the Navy and became a house husband, staying at home to look after the kids. And I got a nursing job, working very long shifts,' Carrie says. They bought their dream house with family close by, but the reality didn't quite match their childhood memories. In particular the level of violent crime worried them and they started looking for a better alternative for their children's future. There was nowhere in England that they particularly wanted to live, so they began to look further afield. Much further. 'We attended a few immigration seminars,' says Carrie. 'Australia seemed too hot and scary, Canada was far too cold, so we started to look very seriously at New Zealand.'

Carrie had never been there before, and the idea of moving to the other side of the world with two young children was quite daunting. But by mid 2005, the idea was gathering pace. Carrie applied for a job as an emergency nurse in Wellington; she was interviewed over the phone and got the job. 'I was pretty experienced and well qualified by then, and nursing skills are transferable all over the world.' From that moment the paperwork took over. Residency visas, medical clearances, contracts of sale on the house. Ian flew over to Wellington on his own and spent a couple of weeks looking for places to live, while Carrie stayed in Sunderland organising the move. 'I spent a lot of time worrying about the details,' she admits. 'I was hugely anxious at that time because we didn't know what anything was going to be like, where we would live, whether we'd make friends. It was all so alien.' This tendency to worry had begun in childhood. 'I think it came from my upbringing; Mum and Nan were worriers, always thinking of the worst possibilities that could happen,' Carrie says.

However, everything was progressing smoothly with the move. Then, just twelve weeks before they were due to leave for New Zealand, Carrie's optic neuritis came back for a third time. 'I was working very hard at the time, doing night shift, and trying to get all the paperwork finalised,' Carrie remembers. 'I started getting symptoms in my right eye again, and I actually had to stop working for a week.' This time, when Carrie consulted her GP, he was the first person in seven years to suggest there might be something more serious than optic neuritis going on. Right on the brink of a dramatic life-changing move, this was the last thing Carrie wanted to hear.

Still, she followed up on his concern, even paying to see a neurologist to avoid the long wait. 'He actually told me that it was quite likely that I had MS,' says Carrie. 'He said that I should forget all about this emigrating malarkey, stay at home close to my family, and be prepared for the inevitable.'

Carrie responded with a mixture of defiance and denial. 'It wasn't a confirmed diagnosis at that point, just a likely one,' she says. 'So on one level I didn't react as if I actually had MS.' After that her stubborn nature kicked in. 'I have never been very good at being told what to do, so once again I thought I'm going to prove the neurologist wrong. I was really very positive; I just knew we had to stick to our plans and not let it stop us from doing what was right for our family,' she says. 'And there were lots of fingers crossed, hoping everything was going to turn out okay.'

Carrie, Ian and the kids arrived in New Zealand in January 2006. They rented a house and found a school for Emily and a nursery for Adam. 'I started working permanent part-time night shift, so that I could look after the kids as well,' remembers Carrie. 'And Ian started working full time as a Sky TV installer, running his own business.' Life was hectic, and there weren't really enough hours in the day for Carrie and Ian to cope with their various responsibilities with work and family. To add to the chaos, they decided to buy a big old house that needed renovating. 'We saw this beautiful 1910 villa that had a really great feel about it,' says Carrie. 'At first Ian said no way, it would be a disaster, but in the end I convinced him it would be a good idea.' In between her shift work at Wellington Hospital and caring for the kids, Carrie began organising plasterers, tilers and painters to come and work on the property that would one day become their home. 'It was a really busy time, but we just threw ourselves into our new lives.'

Everything went well for about nine months. Then one October morning, Carrie was standing at the kitchen sink with her hands poised above the soapy water ready to wash the dishes. 'I put my hands in, and it felt like they had been immersed in ice, even though I knew the water was warm,' she says. Later she noticed a strange feeling in her knee, as if there was an extra bone in her leg and it was made of wood. 'I just dismissed it, put it to the back of my mind,' she admits. Her new life in New Zealand didn't have space for MS.

But before long something happened that was impossible to ignore, and the diagnosis she'd been hiding from for so long finally arrived home. The catalyst was an unpleasant incident at work. As sometimes happens in emergency departments, Carrie was assaulted by a patient and knocked unconscious. 'I was hurt, but it was more a case of a bruised and battered ego than any lasting damage,' she says. However, while taking a few days off work to recover, Carrie's lingering sensory symptoms got noticeably and dramatically worse. 'Within days my legs, arms, speech and vision all started to be affected,' she remembers. 'It got so that I couldn't tie a shoelace or brush my hair.'

In the back of her mind Carrie knew what the problem was, but she just couldn't bring herself to admit it, continuing with the denial that had served her well so far. 'Once you acknowledge that you have MS then you have to deal with it, and I wasn't ready to do that,' she explains. Nevertheless, Carrie kept an appointment with a neurologist, went for an MRI, saw all the lesions in her brain and spinal cord, and was told categorically that she had MS. Despite all the warning signs, the actual diagnosis came as a huge shock. 'I was absolutely devastated. I felt like I'd been hit by a truck,' she says. 'No-one had ever sat there and told me for certain that MS was the problem.'

There is no good time for a diagnosis of MS, but the timing seemed particularly cruel. 'Things had just started to go well for us,' Carrie says. 'Ian had his business up and running and the kids were just getting settled.'

Carrie spent many hours crying to herself and to Ian, worrying about what would happen if she became disabled and unable to look after the family. Her anxious mind considered all the terrible possibilities, even down to the fine detail of what kind of wheelchair she might need and how their house would have to be adapted for disability. Now living thousands of miles away from her parents and most of her friends, it was a very lonely and frightening time.

'Apart from Ian and one close friend, I didn't share my news with anyone,' she says. 'People at work thought I was still recovering from the assault, that I was reluctant to return because of what happened.' That would have been understandable, but the truth was far worse: she was in the middle of a massive MS relapse. It took four weeks, and three days of steroids, for her symptoms to begin to subside, though fatigue remained a major problem. Carrie returned to work and eventually had to tell her manager about the diagnosis. He responded compassionately, but said, 'Oh my, you'll have to move back to England—how will you ever manage on your own over here?' Carrie's fighting spirit again took over. 'I knew there was nothing to move back for, and I knew that we would have to survive on our own, somehow,' she adds.

Still, things couldn't continue as they had been, with Carrie working permanent night shifts, looking after the kids during the day, and organising house renovations in her spare time. She arranged to swap to day shifts, and after a while got a part-time job as a nurse educator, as she had been once before in England. On her neurologist's advice she also started taking a weekly injection of interferon to reduce further relapses. The side effects were very unpleasant for the first twelve weeks, but after that they settled down. At the time, Carrie thought it was the only thing she could do to combat the inevitable progression of MS. 'It seemed like a small price to pay for hopefully staying well,' she reflects.

But overall Carrie's outlook was bleak. 'I was really terrified and I remember asking my neurologist to just give me another ten or fifteen years use of my legs so I could look after the kids until they were independent,' she says. 'He said if I was lucky I would get that long,' she remembers. 'It didn't seem very positive.'

Carrie continued to worry about how Ian and the kids would manage without her. There was the financial strain of being a co-breadwinner, the cost of education and medical expenses, and the reduced social security in New Zealand compared to England. 'It was a huge panic and I have memories of real depression around that time. I didn't need medication for it, but everything felt terribly gloomy and I certainly started confiding in a few friends to get more support,' she says. Through the depression, however, Carrie slowly started to think that there must be something she could do about her situation. 'With all illnesses there is always something you can do that affects your experience; I knew there must be something out there, even though I hadn't found it yet,' she explains.

As her mood improved, she started searching the internet and ordered nearly a dozen textbooks on MS in her hunt for answers. When they arrived in the mail she read them avidly, jotting down anything that might be useful. There wasn't much. It was mostly doom and gloom—lists of symptoms, likely time to disability, and ways of coping with the many unpleasant aspects of the disease. 'I used to wake up every morning and wonder which bits of me were going to stop working,' Carrie recalls. After several weeks the pile of unread books had been reduced to just one or two. One afternoon Carrie picked up Professor George Jelinek's *Taking Control of Multiple Sclerosis* and opened the cover. She found the scientific recommendations extremely convincing. 'I was gripped from the first chapter; it was easy to read and it made absolute sense,' she says. 'It gave me a real feeling of hope and made me think positively for the first time. By doing a few fairly simple things that were not at all alternative, I realised I could affect the way this disease progressed.'

The arrival of hope at last enabled some positive action. For the first few days Carrie inspected every single food label she came across, in her pantry and on supermarket shelves. 'I just wanted to see what we were actually eating,' she says. 'We thought we were eating relatively healthy food, but I soon realised we were not.' The whole family had been eating a lot of meat—particularly red meat—and not enough fruit and vegetables. 'I wouldn't say it was a bad diet, but I didn't really think about what I was putting into my mouth,' Carrie explains. 'The kids ate better than I did, and I came to see just how much hidden sugar and fat there was in a lot of the food we ate.'

Sensing that it might be hard to convert the entire family to a wholefood, plant-based diet plus seafood, Carrie concentrated on herself first, cutting out all meat and dairy, which had made up a large part of her diet in the past. 'A lot of the things I started eating, like tofu and even fish, were really not that popular with the others,' confesses Carrie. 'It was very hard to find a balance of what we could all eat, so we compromised and only occasionally all ate together.'

The one thing Carrie would not compromise on was her own eating plan, which she began to see as a clear path to future health. 'I'd seen the evidence and I knew I'd be stupid not to do it,' she remembers. 'How would I feel in five years time if I didn't make these changes and my MS got worse?' she says. 'I was pretty determined.'

At that time her emotional health was still worse than her physical health. Some of the gloom was starting to lift, but Carrie continued to worry about the future. 'None of this seemed fair on the kids. Your mum should be there to look after you and I didn't want my kids to have to look after me.'

Hoping to find some emotional support among like-minded people, Carrie decided to attend a residential MS retreat. Here she found an outlet for many of her deepest fears—things that until then she had only shared with a handful of people. 'I found it to be a place of great emotional healing,' she recalls. 'It was very important for me to be able to share those feelings in a safe environment. Everyone really understood how I felt and it was like a massive weight being lifted.'

Returning to her life in Wellington, Carrie made time for some of the meditation techniques she had learned at the retreat. 'I had never meditated before and I found it quite difficult, though I did enjoy it,' she says. She also managed to get her vitamin D levels checked and, finding they were rather low, started supplementing.

After just a few short weeks, Carrie realised she had brought something else back from the retreat as well. 'I found that my optimism was starting to grow,' she recalls. 'I think it was because I had met so many people who had gone through similar experiences, and I saw their positivity and how they coped with it.' Carrie realised that getting through the diagnosis of MS was going to be a full-time job. 'I knew I would need a positive outlook to survive, and there was no time for doom and gloom,' she says.

Her mood then received another boost when the fatigue she had been battling for the past eight years started to lift. 'I found I had a new level of energy that I hadn't had for a very long time,' Carrie says. Her fatigue had actually been very debilitating, though not constant, often requiring her to lie down or even sleep in the afternoons. For years she had put it down to the demands of motherhood and nursing, but now she realised that it was very much a part of having MS. 'The fatigue disappeared very quickly and I really believed that it was because the food I was eating was healthier and more energising,' she explains. 'I was juicing a lot too—carrot, beetroot, celery. And I was careful about how I cooked food, grilling fish instead of frying it and watching the kind of oil I used.'

As Carrie was able to do more, running her day-to-day life gradually became easier. 'I started going to the gym and making that a regular part of my lifestyle, though when I got hot it made my symptoms worse,' she remembers. 'To begin with I couldn't stay on the treadmill very long, but eventually I built it up so I could run for four kilometres [two and a half miles] without a problem.'

She also made time to volunteer in the community, becoming involved in the Wellington MS society. 'The field workers were very supportive of making lifestyle changes, especially around diet,' Carrie says. 'I felt there was a lot of understanding there and I really found it helpful.' At the start Carrie just attended meetings, getting to understand the organisation. Later she became a very active committee member.

'I think it helped to maintain my positivity because we really felt we were making a difference,' she adds. 'Luckily everyone was on the same page as me.' Over the years Carrie became secretary and later vice-president of the society, a position she still holds today. 'It's quite overwhelming when you see how much work is being done, and it helped me to look at the bigger picture rather than just at my own situation,' she says.

By 2009 Carrie was easily managing her three day a week job as a nurse educator, exercising regularly, looking after Emily and Adam, and carrying out her volunteer role with the MS society. When a few extra hours of work as a CPR (cardiopulmonary resuscitation) educator were offered at the hospital, she decided she was ready for the challenge. Everything continued to go well. Over the coming months Carrie gradually took on more and more hours until eventually, by 2010, she was working the equivalent of a full-time job again. 'Work has always been a really rewarding part of my life,' she says. 'When I was first diagnosed with MS I didn't think I'd ever get to the point when I'd be able to work more than a few days a week,' she admits. 'Getting back to full-time functioning has been incredibly important to me.'

It isn't only the number of paid hours that have increased over the years, but also the amount of responsibility. 'I now work as a full-time resuscitation officer for the local district health board,' Carrie says. 'That is a very busy job with a lot of responsibility.

I'm managing a team and we have 3500 employees who all need to be current in CPR.'

Every time Carrie has upped her workload, she has assessed her health and considered how it could affect her ability to do the job. 'I don't want to let people down by taking on too much,' she explains. It's a throwback to the constant fear that used to plague her—the thought that the next relapse might be just around the corner, stopping her from working and looking after the children. 'It took a couple of years for that continual fear to go away,' she recalls. 'I used to wake up thinking about it every day, but now it is very much at the back of my mind.' The only time it surfaces is when she takes on something new. 'I still think gosh, can I really do this?' she muses. The answer is usually yes, and Carrie's life is much richer as a result.

Carrie has noticed that she now deals with stress in a far healthier way. 'Every relapse I've had has been around a very stressful time in my life,' she says. 'I don't experience stress the way I used to because I am much more aware of it and conscious of my reactions to events.' She is also very mindful of the way stress affected her negatively as a child. 'I really felt under pressure to achieve and it has made me think about the way I talk to my own kids,' she admits. 'I try not to exert any pressure over their future; I just want them to be happy, go with the flow and they'll get there in the end.'

Carrie says she now gets far more enjoyment out of life, takes more risks and acts more spontaneously. On a family holiday in Auckland a couple of years ago, she surprised everyone by announcing that she was going to bungee jump off the Sky Tower. 'After my second jump the kids were begging me not to do it again!' she laughs.

Now aged 43, it is six years since Carrie's last relapse and fourteen years since MS first entered her life. 'When I started making lifestyle changes I remember wondering how on earth I was ever going to make it to three years,' she says. 'It felt like a real celebration when I got to five years without a relapse, knowing it can be done.'

Carrie has a vision of retiring a little early and enjoying her late fifties and sixties. For many people with MS, that is precisely the period in their lives when they are most adversely affected by the illness. But Carrie no longer expects that to happen to her. 'Once the kids have grown up, we've talked about running a bed-and-breakfast or a homestay out in the country,' she says. 'I haven't even thought about MS in those plans—it just doesn't feature in my thoughts at all. When I was diagnosed I was in such a bleak place,' she remembers. 'But I got through that and I've become well again.'

Carrie Philliskirk still notices occasional, fleeting sensory symptoms in her arms and legs, and occasional fatigue, but nothing else. She has no disability, and doesn't expect to develop any. Carrie's determination has translated into real confidence in herself, and in her future; she knows she will be well for a long time to come.

7

A HARD-FOUGHT BATTLE FOR KNOWLEDGE

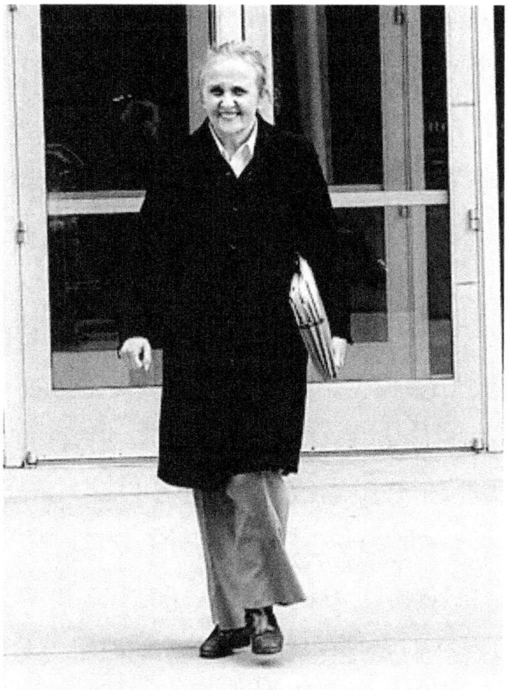

REBECCA HOOVER

Minnesota shapes its people. Perhaps it's the harsh north American climate with its freezing winters, scorching summers and frequent tornadoes. Or the wilderness with its vast lakes and forests populated by bears. Whatever the reason, Minnesotans pride themselves on being tough, practical and down to earth. Rebecca Hoover is no exception.

Rebecca was born on a small dairy farm in the north-west of the state in 1949. This was a time before the large-scale use of pesticides, a time when most food was grown organically, and no-one's dinner came out of a packet. It was a time of great poverty but also of great happiness. The middle one of five children, Rebecca grew up close to nature, spending her summers swimming in the nearby lake with her older sisters and younger brothers. 'The environment was really abundant. Whenever we went fishing we'd always catch something worth eating in less than an hour. We really had a wonderful life despite being cash-poor.'

Her father worked as a sharecropper, ploughing fields and milking cows until Rebecca was eight years old. Then the family moved off the farm and into a nearby small town of around 100 people. From that time her father worked as a carpenter and her mother did odd jobs to make ends meet. Every summer the family used to grow a huge organic vegetable garden. But the winters were harsh.

'The house I grew up in had no indoor plumbing, so even in the middle of winter when it was minus 40 degrees Celsius (minus 40 degrees Fahrenheit) we had to go to an outhouse to use the bathroom,' Rebecca remembers. 'For toilet paper, we usually used old newspapers. That is what we could afford.'

The town's school was a one-room schoolhouse which catered to 25 children of different ages, all in a single classroom. The teachers were excellent, but the facilities were primitive, with no running water or flushing toilet. 'It was basic,' Rebecca says, 'but it was also an incredibly tight-knit community. I still feel a very strong emotional bond with the people I went to school with all these decades later.'

As a child Rebecca was carefree, extroverted and intelligent. By the time she left high school she was ready to take on the world. 'Here I was, a bright one—I thought nothing could ever go wrong for me. I'd figured out I was invincible by the time I was seventeen and I stayed that way right up until I was 41 years old and got diagnosed with multiple sclerosis.'

During those intervening years she gradually moved away from the natural abundance she'd enjoyed in childhood, towards a less healthy, more manufactured and more toxic lifestyle. Not that it seemed that way to her at the time. Outwardly she met academic, professional and social challenges head-on, never doubting that her body would keep going forever.

On leaving school she enrolled at the University of Minnesota. For a few years Rebecca alternated between study and work before finally completing her degree to great acclaim, being awarded a university-wide medal for academic excellence and community service. She returned to the university to teach for a while and pursued a career in IT management, programming and website design. She joined groups such as the Association for Computing Machinery, finding stimulation and interest among such intellectual company.

This was the late 1970s and 1980s, a time when women were becoming part of the political landscape of America. Socially progressive and pioneering, Rebecca was part of that scene, and she found the smoking habit she'd picked up after leaving school fitted in perfectly. 'All the smart politicians were smoking like crazy. I was young and very involved in politics and everybody smoked.'

Rebecca's diet had taken a turn for the worse as well. Her professional status meant she was able to afford the processed food that was arriving on supermarket shelves, and she turned her back on the simple, wholesome nutrition of her childhood.

'At that time I had the unhealthiest lifestyle of all my siblings. Ironically, I thought of myself as intelligent, but my lifestyle was the least healthy of my siblings,' she admits.

Without realising it, Rebecca was accumulating many of the risk factors associated with MS: smoking, a high saturated-fat diet, and low vitamin D. 'Unfortunately for me at that time it was quite popular to stay out of the sun because it caused wrinkles,' she says. Today Rebecca finds that idea hilariously funny, but back then she took it very seriously. 'Wrinkles,' she laughs, 'I didn't want that happening to me!' Of course, what actually happened was far worse than wrinkles.

In the early 1990s Rebecca was living an independent life in Minneapolis–Saint Paul. Socially gregarious and extroverted she was active in the community, on the board of directors for non-profit organisations, still with an eye on politics, enjoying a diverse and challenging working life. She worked as an IT and financial systems consultant, and she arranged her busy social life around contracts, including some with fairly influential clients. Nothing could go wrong. 'I had the most reckless attitude that nothing bad was ever going to happen to me. I didn't bother eating healthy food—that was for little people,' she laughs. 'I wonder how many other people have the same kind of hubris?'

Then everything changed one year in spring. After that she didn't feel invincible anymore.

It was April 1991 when the phone rang one morning in Rebecca's apartment. Getting up to answer it, she could see the first new growth of leaves appearing on the trees outside. She talked to her client for a while before walking slowly back to the kitchen. As she sat down again she became aware of an odd sensation in her left foot, as if it had gone to sleep. She rubbed it, hoping to bring her foot back to life, but the numbness and tingling remained. A few days later the strange sensation was still there.

'I went to the doctor and told him that my foot had gone to sleep. He said, "Don't worry, that happens to a lot of people," so I went away.

'Then my whole leg went to sleep, so I went back and saw a different doctor at the same clinic and told her there was something wrong with my leg. She said, "Don't worry, that really happens to a lot of people for all sorts of reasons," so I went away again,' Rebecca remembers.

'Then it happened in my other foot as well, but the doctor kept telling me not to worry about it.'

Finally one day Rebecca stood up and just fell straight over, spraining her ankle quite badly in the process. 'I went back to the clinic again and said, "I really think there's something wrong," and a doctor finally sent me to a neurologist.'

The subsequent MRI showed up three relatively large lesions. One of these was on Rebecca's spine, causing the weakness and numbness in her legs. The diagnosis of MS came quickly afterwards.

Perhaps it was just the characteristic Minnesotan toughness, but that first neurologist really played down the impact MS was likely to have, suggesting that Rebecca should remain optimistic. No pharmaceutical drugs were available yet, nor did he advocate any diet or lifestyle changes. Still, his attitude was that she should remain hopeful and positive. 'I see a lot of people with MS and I think you should be optimistic,' he told her, adding, 'and believe me I'm very glad you don't have a brain tumour.' Rebecca is now very grateful for his positive approach, though at the time she found his advice impossible to follow.

'Being diagnosed was truly one of the most horrible times in my life. I felt so weak and so very scared. I thought I was going to have all sorts of physical problems and I imagined that I was losing everything, and that no-one would like me when I became disabled,' she admits.

Her view of MS as a disease came partly from the information being distributed by the MS societies, but also from an experience she had while still at high school. In her final year Rebecca had worked at a small nursing home. One of the residents had MS and Rebecca could still picture her sitting in her wheelchair with a little potty underneath. 'It seemed like a pretty dismal existence for her, so when I found out that I had MS the image of this lady came straight into my mind.'

Rebecca collected as much information as possible about the disease. She looked up lists of symptoms to prepare herself for what might happen. She cried a lot. 'I was very depressed and pessimistic about the future. Everything that was written on MS was just so doggone gloomy that it was difficult to have much hope at all,' she says.

'The most optimistic thing was not how to have a full and healthy life, but how you can improve your bowel and bladder problems by wearing adult diapers. So it was pretty hard to even look for things that could make me better. The paradigm was not about getting well—it was about coping with illness.'

As it turned out Rebecca was right to be afraid of the future. There were going to be some very tough times ahead.

The diagnosis brought fear and uncertainty into her life for the first time, but Rebecca tried hard to carry on as normal, attempting to keep the images of wheelchairs and potties at bay. That proved very difficult.

For several months her feet and legs remained weak and numb. Stairs became hard to navigate and her energy was low. She had to cut back on some of her social engagements, opting to stand down as a board member for community organisations. This withdrawal from society only made her feel worse, not better.

'I didn't want to go advertising to the world that I had MS, so I only confided in a very few close friends and relatives, and I never talked about it at work. I didn't think I could count on getting much support,' she says.

Luckily, Rebecca's work at the time was being done largely from home. As an IT consultant she was able to move her office into the bedroom and operate successfully with limited mobility. Her neurologist recommended bed rest for the relapse, something she took very literally. For months she continued to work this way, feigning health when she needed to meet clients, working from her bed whenever possible. Slowly her symptoms began to improve.

After six months she found that her legs had completely recovered. No more numbness, no more weakness, no more tingling. And her energy levels were back to normal too. Just the awful fear remained, that this was all going to end badly.

Then the following year, just as the leaves were reappearing on the Minnesotan trees, she had her second relapse. Again it affected her legs. Again she took to her bed. Weakness meant that she sometimes fell forwards when walking up stairs, though she didn't get injured. It was a tiring and slow recovery, and this time it wasn't a full recovery. Little patches of numbness remained, and Rebecca could tell that overall her strength and energy had been compromised. She used to enjoy running before being diagnosed with MS; now she found she only had the strength for walking, and even then the distances she could walk were getting shorter and shorter.

By the mid 1990s her condition had deteriorated quite considerably. Every year—usually in the spring—she would get renewed problems with her legs. But now some other symptoms had started to creep in as well, the most upsetting of these being a loss of bladder and bowel control. Not a total loss, but enough to make Rebecca constantly on edge whenever she was in public, afraid of being caught out and having an embarrassing accident. During relapses her mobility was severely affected and she was only able to walk 20 metres (22 yards) at the most, and even then she sometimes needed a cane. Driving was difficult at times because of the numbness in her feet, but she managed to keep her car.

Depressed about the future, she nevertheless tried to make the best of the situation, and looked for ways to let her former confident self shine through. 'I went out and bought the cutest cane I could find—a wonderful cane with an eagle's head on the top,' she says. 'And I started investigating scooters, trying to find one that was really sexy. I just thought by God, if I'm going to be disabled then I want to look good while I'm doing it,' she laughs.

In truth, though, she was still hiding her relapses and times of increasing disability from almost everyone. By now it was 1996 and Rebecca was working as a project manager. She spent a lot of time in meetings, sitting down, being careful to stay close to bathrooms because of her poor bowel and bladder control. When the walk from the car park became too much for her to cope with, even with a cane, she applied for a disabled parking permit, but downplayed her walking difficulties.

'I was very careful to avoid creating the impression of disability. I had to be sneaky. Using the disabled permit I could park close to my office, and that meant I didn't need to use a wheelchair at work,' she explains.

'There is a lot of discrimination against people with disability and I was aware of those issues. I thought if I showed my disability that could mean economic disaster or even violence.'

Outside of work, however, Rebecca was needing a wheelchair for long distances during relapses, which meant anything over 20 metres. Shopping trips and airports could no longer always be navigated using her cane.

Then, in 1997, Rebecca had her first attack of optic neuritis and went temporarily blind in one eye. Concerned that she wouldn't be able to drive, she went to her doctor for advice and, pragmatic as ever, he told her: 'Don't worry, you can use your other eye.'

But seven years of relapses had taken their toll. Rebecca wasn't quite ready for the wheelchair with a potty underneath it yet, but her health was becoming increasingly problematic.

Since her diagnosis in 1991, the first pharmaceutical treatments for MS had been approved. Rebecca's neurologist never pushed the idea of drugs and there was, in any case, a waiting list of people clamouring to try them. Names were entered into a lottery, and when Rebecca's was pulled out she thought seriously about her options. 'When Betaseron became available I thought about taking it, but at that time people were talking about the possibility that it might cause genetic mutations,' she recalls. Rebecca's neurologist thought it would be sensible to let other people experiment with the new drug and see what happened.

In 1997 Rebecca was still watching and waiting, fearful of the side effects and quietly sceptical that drugs were the answer. Then one day, not long after her relapse of optic neuritis, she was searching the internet and happened to come across an article on the biomedical literature website PubMed about the neurologist Roy Swank. His remarkable research into a low saturated-fat diet for people with MS had been published some years before in the prestigious British medical journal *The Lancet,* and straight away it appealed to Rebecca's analytical, scientific mind. This, she thought, might be an answer.

'With my academic background I could understand the importance of this research,' she says. 'For the first time I realised that maybe I could have some control over the MS disease process.'

Other people in her life were very sceptical. Her friends indulged her, but they didn't really believe diet and lifestyle could make a difference.

The Swank diet appealed to Rebecca on another level as well. With its emphasis on plant-based wholefoods, it was a link back to the simple nutrition of her childhood, and to her deep love of the environment. Moving away from over-consumption back to a more frugal way of life, she reconnected with something fundamental. 'My lifestyle was so bad for me and so bad for the environment. It was just a little out of sync with what I and the world needed,' she reflects.

Having real hope for the first time since diagnosis, Rebecca put the brochures of mobility scooters to one side and set about transforming her diet. At the time her favourite foods were pizza and fried pork rinds. She cleared out her cupboards, filled her fridge with fresh vegetables, cut back her saturated-fat intake to the suggested 15 grams per day, and waited. 'I had cautious hope at that time, not really daring to believe it could work, but hoping that it might.'

A year later she had another relapse. Optic neuritis again, though not as severe as the previous year. Undeterred, Rebecca stuck to the diet. She still ate some meat, cheese and eggs, but was careful to stay below Dr Swank's recommended daily intake of saturated fat.

Then, while undergoing routine tests with her doctor, Rebecca discovered that she had pre-osteoporosis, an early warning sign that she might suffer from low bone density later in life. Part of the treatment for this condition was to supplement with vitamin D. 'At the time the recommended daily allowance was only 400IU so that is all I was taking,' she recalls.

It wasn't much, but Rebecca believes this simple combination of cutting back on saturated fat and supplementing with vitamin D was enough to halt the relapses. In any case, in the spring of 1999, Rebecca stayed well for the first time that decade. No new problems with her legs, no optic neuritis. 'I was surprised, because I used to get problems every year,' she remembers.

Her surprise gradually turned to wonderment. From that time on, and with the adoption of other lifestyle changes, Rebecca never experienced another relapse, and little by little her mobility, sight and energy all improved. This marked the end of her steady decline with MS, and the start of her very gradual recovery. But it was a slow process, and one that has really only been possible to appreciate in hindsight.

Rebecca describes her return to health as a kind of awakening, but not the kind where you suddenly see a bright light and everything changes. 'It was a hard-fought battle for knowledge, rather than a Road to Damascus kind of event. I didn't ever feel "Wow, I'm getting well"—it really wasn't like that at all,' she says. 'Just gradually and very slowly I started to feel better, but the improvements were all really subtle.'

The first thing Rebecca noticed was an increased sense of touch. For years her feet had lacked sensitivity and she'd been unable to feel the plush carpet as she walked around her home. In 1999, two years after starting the Swank diet, she felt the wonderful sensation of softness between her toes as she pressed her feet down into the bedroom carpet.

As her physical health began to improve, so her mood lifted too. 'What happens to you psychologically when you start making lifestyle improvements is very significant,' she says. 'I had been so pessimistic—sure that MS was going to take over my whole life and I would end up very disabled. But once I started to eat right and add other wellness strategies into my life, my whole outlook changed.'

Gradually Rebecca's working life became easier too. No longer needing to hide her previously increasing disability, she could relax a little more around her colleagues and business associates. She also started to take on some of the community responsibilities she had relinquished at the start of her illness.

With no spring relapse to recover from in 1999, Rebecca's overall health received a real boost. After a while she noticed that she didn't need to use a wheelchair while out shopping anymore. In the years that followed she was able to walk ever-increasing distances, first with her cane and later without it. 'During the 1990s I never really walked more than 800 metres (875 yards) at a time, and that was only between relapses,' she says. 'But by 2003 I was already able to walk for four or five kilometres (two and a half to three miles) at a time.'

One freezing winter's day when the ice and snow lay on the streets of Minneapolis, Rebecca set off briskly down the stairs of her apartment building and out onto the suburban streets of her neighbourhood for her daily walk. No longer needing a cane, she just had her running shoes for support. Halfway round she hit a particularly icy patch and slipped, breaking her ankle in the process. 'That's the last time I used that old wheelchair,' she remembers, though she is adamant that MS played no part in her fall. 'Breaking bones is an industry here in Minnesota in the winter,' she laughs.

In 2004 some more pieces of research-based knowledge were added to Rebecca's recovery plan. The first was strenuous exercise. Already a keen walker, she had been steadily building up her distances over the previous few years. Now she added weightlifting into the regime. 'I was reading the research on weightlifting and resistance training and I discovered that it not only improves your physical fitness, but also your brain capacity.' To begin with Rebecca was lifting very low weights, but felt happy to be able to lift anything at all. Then gradually she built up until she could lift 1800kg (4000lb) over one session. 'The improvements sneaked up on me gradually so I didn't really notice,' she says.

Around the same time Rebecca came across some research from Harvard medical school suggesting that running short intervals is more beneficial than walking or jogging alone. Her fitness allowed her to add this into her exercise plan, walking briskly for 30 minutes before running hard in one-minute bursts, interspersed with walking.

Though her mobility and strength were much improved, in 2004 Rebecca was still having bowel control issues. With a history of chronic diarrhoea that predated her diagnosis of MS, she decided to remove all dairy and gluten from her diet after reading that these foods might be the culprits. The very next day her bowel issues resolved and have never returned.

By 2008 Rebecca's diet and lifestyle plan included a gluten-free, low saturated-fat diet with no dairy and hardly any meat, supplementation with vitamin D and fish oil, and strenuous exercise. And she no longer smoked. Looking back over ten years of gradual improvements she was able to see just how remarkable her recovery had been. 'I realised that I was healthier than I had been in 1991 before I first got diagnosed, and that's a pretty amazing thing,' she reflects. 'Some people make changes and try for a year and decide that it's not working. But you have to try for three, four, five years, and then when you look back you can see the difference,' she adds. 'I think when people realise that recovery can be a subtle process then it gives them hope. Unrealistic expectations can be their worst enemy.'

Rebecca says that patience is important and it pays off. She points out that while individual lesions have come and gone during her life with MS, overall they have reduced in size. 'When I was diagnosed in 1991, the radiologist's report on my brain MRI said the largest lesion was 10mm by 5mm,' she says. 'Nearly two decades later the largest recorded lesion was only 6mm by 5mm, and most of the remaining lesions were very small—only 2mm by 3mm.'

The year of 2008—ten years since her last relapse—marked another turning point for Rebecca. Finally confident that she had reversed the effects of MS, she decided to break her silence about the disease and launch her own informative website, 'The intelligent person's guide to beating MS'. Her increasing age, and increasing health, made her an excellent role model and symbol of hope for other people who were being diagnosed. Drawing on her business background, she pooled her powers of persuasion to create a slightly sassy and naughty website. 'I do get called "Her Naughtiness" by my friends, and I love telling slightly rude jokes,' she laughs.

Rebecca uses humour whenever she can, but her underlying message is practical, straightforward and full of hope: you can beat MS. Part of the inspiration for her website came from the memory of a lady she was introduced to soon after diagnosis. This lady, who was in her 70s, walked with a cane but was otherwise in good health, despite having had MS for many years. 'She told me that MS doesn't have to be so bad, and over all the depressing things she was my one beacon of hope,' Rebecca remembers. 'When I saw how well I was doing using only a lifestyle approach, compared to other people who were taking the drugs for MS, I thought that could provide hope for others too,' she says.

Rebecca Hoover is very keen to point out all the things she did not need to do in order to recover from MS. She did not take steroids or any disease-modifying drugs, she did not have her dental amalgams removed (though she has plenty in her mouth), she did not have bee sting therapy, follow an anti-Candida diet, or have CCSVI (chronic cerebrospinal venous insufficiency) treatment. Soon after diagnosis she began writing a journal, but stopped again almost immediately. 'There are far more interesting people to write about in the world than me,' she laughs. And she has never meditated; hasn't the patience for it. 'Everything I've done has been scientific and measurable,' she says, somewhat unconvinced by the volumes of literature on the health benefits of meditation.

Over the last few years her regime has been tweaked as new research has come into the public domain. When vitamin D became more widely discussed, and high doses were being recommended, Rebecca gradually increased her levels from the minimal supplementation to fairly large doses of 50,000IU every week. After this she noticed another boost to her energy, strength and mood. She also takes a vitamin B [12] supplement twice a week, as she has since 1991, and later experimented with B [6] after some tingling in her toes, which she sensed was not MS related. 'I started researching and found that a B [6] deficiency could cause these symptoms. At first I took too much, which caused more problems, but once I pulled it back the tingling disappeared. Not everything is an MS problem—sometimes it can just be nutritional deficiency,' she explains.

Rebecca also ensures that she gets a minimum of seven hours sleep a night, believing this is essential to health. Remembering her first neurologist's advice, she still uses sleep proactively to prevent illness. 'When I feel a cold or flu coming on I don't resist it—I go to bed and get extra rest. I don't think it's good to push yourself so hard that you cause a flare-up of symptoms. You can avoid that just by having a little commonsense.'

Today Rebecca is heading for retirement age but, as intellectually capable as ever, she shows no signs of slowing down, let alone stopping. She now works a very full-time job in debtor's rights, advocating for people who are at risk of losing their homes and possessions.

'I have an amazingly rich and full life and have been fortunate to work with some wonderful people. I really appreciate the confidence people have in me,' she says.

When Rebecca Hoover was at her most disabled from MS in the 1990s, she seriously wondered if she would live to see retirement. Now aged 62, she is wondering if she can make it to 95, like one of her grandmothers.

She certainly sees her recovery as remarkable, showing that it is possible to halt and reverse MS using diet and lifestyle intervention. Once fearing a future in a wheelchair, she now has a full and active life, with only a few minor symptoms to remind her of the problems she once had. For example, her legs often feel a bit sore, which can be alleviated with stretching exercises, and the skin on her feet seems to burn when she puts on lotion. 'These things are really not a big deal. Most people my age have far greater health problems, while I just have a little soreness—and I'm really not going to complain about that,' she says.

Rebecca is healthier than most of her friends and family, running intervals, lifting weights and eating a fish and plant-based diet. 'I can walk on tiptoe and pretend to be Beyoncé for fifteen minutes,' she laughs, 'while my overweight neighbours who don't have MS and are much younger than me can't do any of those things.

'They are at risk of dying young, and they say at least they're going to die happy—as if you're somehow miserable because you're eating healthy food!'

In fact, as well as improving her health beyond recognition, Rebecca's lifestyle change has brought her closer to the core values she grew up with, and closer to happiness. The simple, frugal life that is now so important to her fits perfectly with the basics of really good nutrition. 'It doesn't have to cost a lot to live ultra healthy. I'm a Minnesotan by golly and I don't believe in anything expensive or snobby,' she says.

Interestingly, the state of Minnesota has one of the highest life expectancies in the US, and some of the people who live the longest are quite impoverished. 'They eat a healthy diet and have great community support, and they just live on and on with very few health problems,' Rebecca says. 'Isn't that interesting—the very diet that makes you well is also the one that is best for the environment? You're really not giving anything up—you're actually getting more, and giving more.'

8

ALL ABOUT LOVE

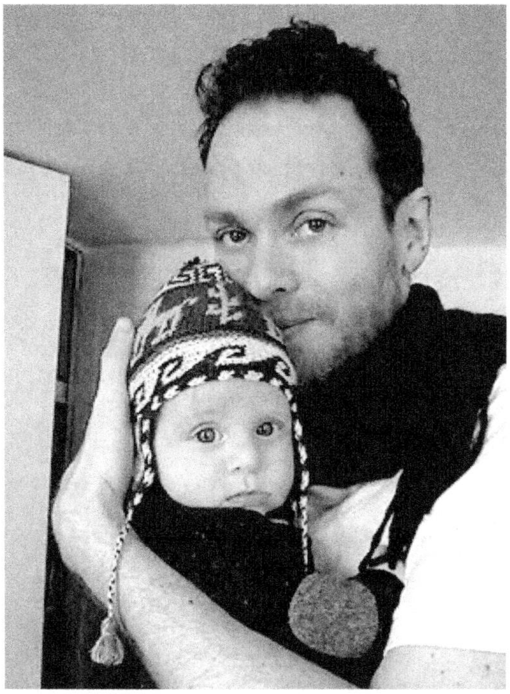

GASPAR HOYOS

Gaspar Hoyos exudes peace. Almost everyone who comes into contact with the 40-year-old flautist notices it—a joyful serenity that seems to seep out of him quite effortlessly. And it's contagious.

It's tempting to assume that such tranquillity has always been part of him, linked to his deep love and passion for music. But actually this is not the case. Before he was diagnosed with multiple sclerosis, Gaspar was a very different man: a brilliant but rather serious and introverted musician. He believes the illness has changed him, for the better.

Gaspar grew up in the Colombian capital Bogotá, the only child of parents who loved classical music but didn't perform it themselves. His dad learned popular songs on the guitar, but it was his parents' classical record collection that he remembers being the main musical influence of his youth. Not that Gaspar played any instruments himself to begin with, apart from the inevitable school recorder. In fact it wasn't until he was fourteen years old that he decided to start taking lessons, although his choice of flute was almost accidental. 'I remember watching the film *Amadeus* about the life of Mozart. That's when I decided I wanted to become a musician,' he says. He told his best friend about his plan, and suggested that they both take violin lessons. 'My friend said, "Oh no, not violin, let's play the flute," and I listened to him because he was my best friend,' says Gaspar. 'So I asked my dad to find me a flute, which was quite difficult in Bogotá at that time. Finally my dad found one, but my friend never got a flute so he never started learning.'

From that moment, music completely dominated the young Colombian's life. He practised incessantly, not because he was told to but because he wanted to. And he advanced incredibly quickly. 'I guess I was gifted—I had a talent for it. Some people used to say that I must have been a flute player in a previous life,' he says with a smile.

Somehow Gaspar completed high school, though he was so in love with music that maths, physics and chemistry meant nothing to him anymore. In 1990 he moved to Ohio to study with a respected flute teacher. He enrolled at a university in Texas, completing his undergraduate degree in 1994. For his Masters degree he chose the New England Conservatory of Music in Boston. Then he set off for Paris, on the trail of another great teacher.

Now part of a European elite group of young musicians, Gaspar did what many of his contemporaries were doing and began entering competitions. And he was very successful. In 1998 he won first prize in Markneukirchen in Germany, and fourth prize in the Jean-Pierre Rampal competition in France. His career was assured.

The following year, at the age of 27, he took the job of principal flautist with the Opéra National de Lorraine in the French town of Nancy, a post he still holds today. The orchestra performs both symphonic concerts and operatic works and has a busy schedule of rehearsals. In addition Gaspar soon found he was in demand as a soloist, accepting invitations to perform with orchestras in America, Japan and Europe. 'You can feel very exposed, and sometimes the concerts would bring quite a lot of stress, especially for the principal flute or as a soloist,' he admits. 'I loved this work, this feeling of performing, but I used to take a lot of the stress home.'

When rehearsals were less than perfect, Gaspar noticed an increasing sense of frustration starting to build up inside him. His love of music had taken him all the way to the top of his profession, but it wasn't always a comfortable place to be. 'When it was not perfect in rehearsals I would get very upset. I knew this feeling was a problem, but I never did anything about it—as if it was normal to be frustrated because things were not perfect,' he says. Gaspar attributes this perfectionism to his rather strict schooling, where lack of attention and bad grades would lead to humiliation. 'I also had the kind of personality that wanted to please others, make everyone happy.'

The frustration that had crept into his musical life featured in his personal life too. His marriage in 2002 to another musician from the orchestra had brought him a son, Esteban, but just two years later the marriage had failed. In 2009 Gaspar and his ex-wife were still caught up in a rather messy and difficult divorce. 'We couldn't find a balance and I felt powerless to do anything about it. I was afraid for our son because he really needed a more stable situation,' says Gaspar. To complicate things further, his new partner, Noémie, was a member of the same orchestra.

In early December 2009, Gaspar and Noémie had enjoyed a pleasant evening having dinner with friends. They didn't share an apartment yet, but they spent a lot of time together. The next morning Gaspar remembers waking up and noticing an unusual pain behind his left ear, and another at the back of his head. The pain was slight but constant, remaining for several days. In time he noticed that his neck and right shoulder had started to go numb. He went to his doctor, who suggested he was suffering from stress. This may have been true, but it wasn't the cause of his increasing symptoms. After Christmas he found that his right thigh was going numb, and finally the symptoms reached a part of him that was vital to his life as a musician—his left hand. Still his doctor maintained it was stress, and no investigations were carried out. By now it was the middle of January and the orchestra was performing Debussy. Gaspar managed to keep playing, but it was getting difficult.

On 23 January, things went downhill very quickly. 'I had trouble walking, and within two days I was taken to hospital. When I got there the only parts of my body that were still working were my eyes, ears, nose, mouth and brain. Everything else had stopped,' Gaspar recalls.

This could have been terrifying for the dedicated musician and father—for a man who until that point had needed everything to be perfect. In fact, what Gaspar Hoyos felt as he lay in his hospital bed was freedom. 'I don't look back on that as a scary time. In a way that was my moment of fortune—from then on I have been free and that is so amazing. I was freed from all the things that I'd attached such importance to, but which don't matter at all.'

In an instant the feelings of frustration, of powerlessness, of perfectionism, just disappeared. They were replaced with love. 'I realised that I had a beautiful family, despite the divorce. I had this great love for my son and this great love for my partner Noémie.'

Gaspar also realised how lucky he was to have music in his life. In a way he had always known that, but he had never felt it so intensely. 'Before that I always believed I had to achieve things in music, to do everything really well. That attitude makes you forget that actually music is love,' he says.

Lying there in the hospital with a body that was no longer working, Gaspar felt that he had two choices: to give up, or to look up and see what was important in life. 'I chose to look up, and all at once I felt peace.'

Emotional freedom began in an instant, but the road to physical freedom was a much harder one to travel. Every day the nurses came and pumped 1.5 grams of steroids into his veins, and every day Gaspar just lay there, unable to move. On the first day he'd been wheeled out for an MRI, but the only doctors he saw were medical students on their rounds. He felt like an animal in a zoo. The diagnosis came on day three of his hospital stay, when the neurologist finally made a ward visit. 'He told me that there were several lesions—one very big one on my brain—and that it looked like multiple sclerosis,' remembers Gaspar. 'He told me my condition was very serious.'

His next visit was from the wheelchair and walking-aid manufacturers, keen to share their brochures with a potential new customer. They horrified Gaspar with their apparent insensitivity and bleak picture of his future. 'These people were talking to me as if I was completely disabled. They showed me a picture of my life that was not very pretty.'

Among the comings and goings of medical staff, however, one person stood out—a young medical student called Philippe, who was kind and optimistic. In contrast to the others, this man had a natural intelligence and great bedside manner. On the fourth day of Gaspar's hospital stay, Philippe entered the room and said, 'Okay, now you're going to walk.' Until then Gaspar had been using a stroller to move even the shortest distance from his bed, and a wheelchair to get outside for some fresh air. The idea of walking seemed ludicrous, but the young medic was encouraging and insistent. 'I remember I was hanging onto the rails around the bed and onto the apparatus that my steroids were hooked on, but he said, "No, I want you to walk on your own," which seemed impossible,' recalls Gaspar. 'But he seemed so sure I could do it that I let go of everything and I walked. This man showed me I could do something that I didn't think I could do.'

The next day Gaspar was allowed to go home. While he had been in hospital Noémie had moved all her belongings out of her own home and into his apartment. She was ready for them to start their new life together, whatever that might mean. 'I was lying there, hardly able to move, and she brought all her things to my place, which is such a beautiful gesture. She was telling me she would be there for me no matter what,' he says.

Despite Gaspar's physical distress, his relationships were maturing. 'I remember Noémie telling me that she felt I was more there for her than I had ever been before—more present,' he says. 'Isn't it funny that when your body is not working at all, other people can actually see you as something more, not less?'

Back in his downtown apartment, he spent the first few days in bed or lying on the couch. When Noémie had to rehearse with the orchestra, other friends came to help out. His body was uncooperative, but the new feeling of peace stayed with Gaspar, pervading all he did. It felt strange when his friends grumbled about having to go out and get jobs done; to him the idea of leaving the apartment was a luxury.

During this time Gaspar made daily phone calls to his mum in Bogotá. She was particularly involved in his journey, not just because she was his mum, but because she also had MS. Unlike her son, however, she had a very mild form of the disease that had only brought three relapses in 40 years. Gaspar found her calm and patient optimism a great source of comfort.

From the moment he returned home, Gaspar began working with a physiotherapist, an inspiring practitioner called Dominique. This was February 2010, and he was finding it very hard to move, let alone play music. Together they worked on picturing the correct motion for walking, teaching him what to do with his recalcitrant legs. On her second visit Dominique brought a walking stick, but it was presented as a temporary measure, rather than something Gaspar would be keeping forever. He accepted it gladly.

'In those early days my son Esteban used to laugh at me when I tried to walk. He'd say, "Oh Daddy, you're walking like a clown!" and then he'd copy me,' remembers Gaspar. This actually provided some light relief. 'I thought it was funny and it made me laugh. Then when I got the stick he told me I was walking like Charlie Chaplin.'

After two and a half weeks, Dominique encouraged Gaspar to venture outside. At first he protested, but she insisted, and together they made it round the block. Then she went on holiday for a week. By the time she returned, Gaspar could no longer walk—MS had struck again, even harder than before.

Back in the hospital, sitting in a wheelchair once more, Gaspar looked up as the neurologist came into the consulting room. Stopping next to the wheelchair, he patted Gaspar on the knee and said, 'Sorry, I think your MS is very aggressive,' before leaving the room. Gaspar was left there pondering his future. 'Sometimes as a patient you listen to these doctors in white coats and it's like they write the script of your life.

Their words can seem like the real truth, and there's nothing you can do about it,' he says.

After a couple of minutes, Gaspar saw the door opening again and Philippe walked in—the young medical student who had previously been so encouraging. His approach was totally different. 'He told me that my future was not written down, that no-one could say for sure that I was going to have a terrible downhill progression,' Gaspar says. When Philippe left the room, Gaspar was filled with a strong feeling that he was going to get better. 'I can't say where that came from, but I think it was my body telling me that the neurologist was wrong and that I would recover.'

At that point Gaspar opted to go home, to take the dose of steroids as an outpatient and to begin his prescribed injections of the disease-modifying drug Rebif. He was tired of the hospital and its doom and gloom predictions.

It would be hard to overestimate the enormity of the task that lay ahead as Gaspar returned to his apartment to begin his journey back to health. This relapse had once again affected his whole body, but this time his arms had curled in on themselves cruelly, and his hands had become claws. Meanwhile his legs had done the opposite, refusing to bend at all, and he had spasticity, tremors and pain.

As an elite musician he had spent tens of thousands of hours honing his skills, training his hands to perform intricate movements with incredible speed and absolute precision. Now they seemed useless.

And it wasn't only his hands and fingers that needed to work well to play music at that level—he also needed a strong chest for breathing, and strong shoulders and arms for holding the flute. These parts of him had been ravaged by MS and his fingers had practically no feeling in them at all.

Still, the freedom that Gaspar had felt at the start of his illness stayed with him, and it was a constant source of encouragement. He wanted to be able to put his new understanding into practice, to create the beauty and love that he now knew music to be. From his years with the orchestra, Gaspar was used to spending many hours painstakingly working through difficult passages of music, repeating tricky phrases until he got them right. Now he applied this technique to his physical rehabilitation.

Soon after he came home from hospital, an interesting parcel arrived in the mail from Colombia. Gaspar's dad had made him a wooden tactile box, filled with objects of varying textures to help bring some feeling back to his damaged hands. Gaspar worked on this tirelessly. To begin with, when he closed his eyes and put his hands on the objects he couldn't feel the difference between a wire brush and a cuddly toy. 'I worked on that so hard that in the end I memorised where all the different things were,' he recalls.

He resumed physiotherapy as soon as Dominique came back from holiday. The first day when he tried to move his legs, it seemed like absolutely nothing was happening. This was very distressing, but Dominique was able to give a glimmer of hope. 'Even in the hardest times she would reassure me,' Gaspar says. 'She would touch my foot all over and look so closely while I tried to move my toes. If she saw just the tiniest bit of movement that was enough.'

Once some movement had returned to his legs, Gaspar relearned how to walk with a cane, going slowly round the block once more. After a couple of weeks his hands had opened up from their claw-like position, but he struggled to perform simple tasks, let alone anything complex or intricate like playing an instrument. 'I remember going to find my flute in its case and I had the hardest time even putting it together. When I tried to hold it up, ready to play, it was like my body didn't understand what to do,' he says.

Now Gaspar started using visualisation to speed up his recovery. This was something that came quite naturally to him, something he didn't need to be taught. In hospital during his first MRI he'd found himself playing Mozart concertos to pass the time inside the tunnel. Later, while lying in his hospital bed, he'd closed his eyes and pictured himself walking up and down the stairs to his apartment.

One afternoon in March, Gaspar was in his kitchen practising a physiotherapy exercise that Dominique had recommended. He was standing on the floor, trying to lift his foot up and put it onto a chair. He tried many times, but it seemed impossible for him to lift it high enough. Then he closed his eyes and imagined himself successfully completing the exercise. When he opened his eyes and tried again, his foot flew straight up in the air, even higher than the chair.

'Doing things in my mind before doing them physically is very important to me. Having an image in my mind about how my body is meant to work is important too,' he explains. For Gaspar, this translated into an image of wellness, of a body working as it is supposed to work. 'For me it was important not to accept my symptoms as something permanent. My body was meant to heal—everyone's body is meant to heal,' he says. 'When you cut yourself, you heal. I really believe in that.'

By April Gaspar's body was indeed healing. He was recovering well from the second attack, and even though he suffered another very small relapse, it only affected his right leg for one week. 'That was the end of my problems—after that it was all recovery,' he says happily.

Gaspar had spent two months working tirelessly on his physical recovery, but his emotional growth was continuing too. In March he began seeing a psychologist, a man who from the start was an important guide and who later became more of a companion on his healing journey. This is where Gaspar started learning about, and talking about, his own emotions for the first time. 'We talked about my painful divorce and he helped me to acknowledge a lot of the emotions I had been feeling. Before that I used to shut down and put everything in a drawer that would not get looked in again,' he recalls.

Gaspar was now much more open to his own feelings, and was enjoying a growing sense of freedom and appreciation for the important things in life. As soon as he regained enough mobility to take his son to school in the mornings, he started delighting in this simple task. Previously it had been a chore, now it was a pleasure. But although his own attitude to life had changed, he realised that many of the people around him had stayed the same. 'I had a hard time understanding other people's bitterness and negativity, and I started to feel frustrated by that,' he says. 'I think once you have been unable to walk you realise that walking is a gift, and it's difficult when other people don't see it that way.'

With the help of his psychologist, Gaspar started using visualisation for emotional as well as physical healing. 'I knew I had this strength in me, this love, and I pictured it coming out of my body and going everywhere,' he explains. 'I know how this mood can be contagious—this peaceful attitude with a gentle smile.' Rather than trying to contradict other people's negativity with words, Gaspar learned to simply give out his own peaceful energy instead. It is this powerful tranquillity that affects everyone he meets, including the psychologist who started him on the journey. 'I could share all my discoveries with him and he listened to it all and even applied it to his own life. At the end of our sessions he would practically thank me as well,' says Gaspar happily.

As spring turned to summer, Gaspar started reading voraciously. His quest for knowledge began with Dr David Servan-Schreiber's *Anti Cancer: A new way of life,* which in turn steered him towards books on healing, meditation, visualisation, nutrition and diet. Soon after his diagnosis he'd read about Dr Roy Swank's research into diet, but he'd had a hard time believing it would work. 'My first reaction was that it was so simple it couldn't possibly be true,' he admits. 'No-one had ever told me about nutrition. I mean, everyone talks about not getting fat, but I never imagined the effect that diet was having on every cell in my body. I really felt angry that no-one had ever explained that,' he adds.

Later, coming across Professor George Jelinek's *Overcoming Multiple Sclerosis* encouraged Gaspar to take another look at Dr Swank's research. 'Jelinek takes you by the hand and shows you that Swank's writings are very serious,' he says. 'Once I realised how important the Swank research was I had something to hang on to—I had faith that this diet would help me to live a normal, long and healthy life.'

Gaspar's typically French diet, high in cheese, meat and yoghurt, was swapped for the wholefood, plant-based diet that was being recommended. He also began supplementing with vitamin D, quite a necessity after so many years spent indoors rehearsing with the orchestra.

Gaspar's reading exposed him to many of the modern pioneers of healing: Deepak Chopra, Bernie Siegel, and also Émile Coué, one of the founders of hypnotherapy. After reading Coué's *Self Mastery Through Conscious Autosuggestion,* Gaspar decided to try hypnotherapy for himself. 'It really played a huge part in my whole recovery,' he says.

At first Gaspar used it to calm his racing mind. 'I used to have 50,000 thoughts going through my mind every day. The brain is crazy—it talks nonsense all day long,' he says. The next thing he did under hypnosis was to reprogram his brain to stop negative images being created. At that time, so soon after two debilitating relapses, frightening images of the future would often come into his head. Images of him sitting in a wheelchair, disabled, alone, unable to play music. Working with Fabrice, his hypnotherapist, he put together what he calls an 'image-destroying machine' to remove those negative pictures. 'But that wasn't enough,' Gaspar explains, 'because I had to replace them with positive images as well.'

He replaced the lonely wheelchair image with a happy picture of himself running around playing with his son. 'In the beginning that wheelchair image would come 100 times a day, but when you catch that thought you can replace it every time with the new image,' he explains. 'After just one week, the wheelchair stopped coming,' he says. 'It's really not difficult to do—you just have to believe in it.'

At this point meditation also became a strong tool in the healing process as Gaspar replaced fear with joy and beauty. 'I was no longer lying there imprisoned by negative thoughts; in my mind I was healing all the time,' he says.

As Gaspar's hands, arms and fingers regained strength and mobility, he used visualisation to enhance his flute playing. At first he just played scales in his mind, then he worked his fingers over difficult technical passages. One day, quite early on in his musical recovery, he closed his eyes and played through Bach's entire Sonata in E Major. It was a piece of music he knew well, and one that included particularly difficult fingering for him as it relied heavily on the little finger of his left hand. After he played the sonata in his mind, Gaspar went for a sleep. 'When I woke up I got out my flute and was able to play the whole piece. I guess I played it through a little stumbling, but it really felt like a miracle,' he says.

From then on Gaspar continued to play every day—not just orchestral pieces as before, but other styles of music that he now found helpful and uplifting. 'I was no longer playing the music that everybody plays for the competitions, I was playing music that spoke to my heart,' he says. He was particularly drawn to the work of his good friend Gary Schocker. 'His music is full of energy and love; it is very human music. There were some pieces of his that I really wanted to play because they are full of emotion. I found that very helpful in the recovery of my attitude towards playing.'

For the next two months Gaspar continued to play music every day and his body continued to recover. By June 2010, just four months after his first relapse, he was able to return full time to his position as principal flute with the orchestra. His sheer passion for music, combined with all the healing techniques he could muster, had taken his crippled hands and coaxed them back to concert standard.

When Gaspar returned to the orchestra, it was paradoxically both easier and harder for him. Easier because he was now playing purely for love. Harder because, to begin with, his fingers didn't move quite as smoothly as before. Not that anyone noticed—what they did notice was a renewed energy in his playing, and the love and emotion coming through. 'People have said that my playing is different now, and they mean that in a positive way,' Gaspar says. 'When you're only worried about perfection, when you're showing off, then you completely forget the beauty of the music and what it's all about. When you base your music-making on emotions it is so simple and beautiful, and that's why it's only pleasure for me now.'

By 2011 Gaspar was enjoying his musical life far more than ever before. Technically he was as good as ever, but he now had an added strength, a greater emotional connection with the music. His CD of Bach sonatas was released and he once again started performing as a soloist with leading orchestras around the world.

'I was asked to play a very challenging piece with the Simon Bolivar orchestra in Venezuela,' he says. 'Had it been any other orchestra there's no way I would have accepted. I went because these guys use music to give hope to children, to take them out of their daily reality, which is incredible. They play music at the highest possible level and are completely in love with what they do.'

Gaspar had a great experience and enjoyed the chance to teach while he was there. 'I think maybe I was looking for people who understand that it is a gift to be able to make music,' he says.

If Gaspar's musical life was going well, his personal life was going even better. In September that year he was blessed with what he calls 'a miraculous gift of life' when Noémie gave birth to their son Tobias. 'When I was diagnosed with aggressive MS, the neurologist was talking about very harsh treatments,' he says. 'The side effects included not being able to have children, which was a very hard thing to hear. I'm so glad I didn't need to take them, but it still felt like a miracle when Tobias was born.'

In April 2012, two years after diagnosis, Gaspar was called back to the hospital for a routine MRI. The last time he'd seen his neurologist, Gaspar had been sitting in a wheelchair and his prognosis was very bad. Two years later, things looked rather different. This time he walked to the appointment, setting off briskly down the steps from his apartment into the streets of the old part of town. He was feeling positive about the MRI, but even he was unprepared for what happened next.

'I was expecting to be told that there were no new lesions—I really had a sense that everything was going well,' he says. But when Gaspar walked into the consulting room, the neurologist was staring at the computer screen with an incredulous look on his face. Without even saying good morning, he pointed to the screen and asked Gaspar what he could see. 'I stared at the screen for a long time and I couldn't see any of the white or grey spots anymore—it seemed totally clear of lesions.' Then the neurologist got very excited, describing it as 'perfect' and 'amazing' and urging Gaspar to celebrate this incredible result. 'He actually told me that based on this scan he would not be able to make a diagnosis of multiple sclerosis. Even the big lesion on my brain had disappeared.'

Gaspar walked back to his apartment with tears of joy streaming down his face. 'I never expected that. It was so encouraging to see that everything I was doing was working. This whole package of healing—this stubborn attitude of keeping the body in balance with positive thoughts and the right diet—it was all working.'

When Gaspar tries to sum up exactly what healing means to him, the word that comes to mind is love.

'From the very beginning, when I found freedom, I realised I had been looking at life from the wrong angle,' he says. 'I was trying to be productive and looking for recognition when actually I had something more important that was right next to me,' he explains.

'My conclusion is really that love is the most important thing,' he says. 'So it's love for my family, love for my healers, and love for music. It's all love and it's all so simple.'

9

FINDING AUTHENTICITY

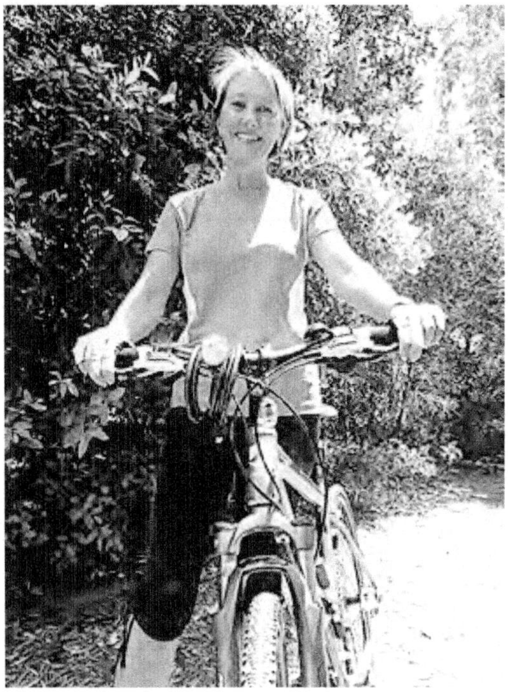

MEGAN SWAN

Megan Swan was riding horses before she was out of nappies. Helped up by her parents, tucked in behind one of her four older sisters as she rode around the huge sheep station her father managed on the east coast of New Zealand. It wasn't long before she graduated to a little pony of her own. The property—Huiarua Station at the foothills of Mount Hikurangi—is the first place in the world to see the sun come up each day, and Megan's days often started early enough to see it. Her childhood was spent outdoors, simple and carefree, and always around horses. 'The station was 23,000 acres (9308 hectares), and it was long and narrow so there were working yards at mid points across it,' says Megan. 'There were around 400 horses there altogether.'

The property was very remote, but as the largest sheep station in the area it created its own community. The eight families of stockmen and fencers, mostly from a Maori background, provided enough children for a small school. Megan, her sisters, plus some children from neighbouring stations joined them for their education, and the station's schoolteacher lived with the shepherds in the single working men's quarters. Each shepherd had around a dozen horses, and right across the property the main method of transport was on horseback. Riding wasn't just a necessity, it was also great fun and formed the backbone of the isolated community's social life. 'There were always competitions,' remembers Megan. 'Potato races, jumping and other fun events, all done on horseback. Horse sports and dog trials were the social focus for the whole area, and groups came from all around to compete,' she says. At this early stage the riding competitions were just for fun. 'All ages and stages could do it,' says Megan. 'Mums and dads, children—everybody was on horses.'

When she reached high school Megan followed her sisters to boarding school in Auckland, but every holiday brought her back home to the horses. 'As we got older we used to hang out with the shepherds on our horses, pretending to work,' she laughs. 'We were quite useful really—we used to get sent ahead to open gates when they were mustering.'

It was at this time that Megan started getting interested in competitive horseriding, a hobby that continued when the family moved off the station and into the town of Gisborne. 'Dad ended up supervising several big stations, so we moved into town so he could be more centrally located to these stations,' she explains.

With riding and showjumping dominating her young life, Megan was not interested in staying on at school. She left as soon as she could at the age of sixteen, getting a job as a teller in the local bank. 'It was owned by Lloyds at the time, with the black stallion logo,' she remembers, 'so everyone used to joke that I even had horses in my work.'

While her spare time was spent riding, her dreams were filled with thoughts of travel. Megan had attended high school with the daughters of Sir Edmund Hillary, and whenever he visited the school he would talk about his travels and adventures on Mount Everest. 'He inspired me to want to travel,' says Megan. 'He made me see there was an amazing world out there.'

For a few years Megan worked two jobs, doubling as a waitress in the evenings to earn extra money so she could go travelling. By the age of 20 she had saved enough money to leave Gisborne and head overseas. The first place she went was Nepal. 'I went with a girlfriend as part of a round-the-world trip, and we visited the Everest Base Camp where all the expeditions left from.' While she was there, however, Megan experienced a major health event and ended up flying home early.

'I suddenly got numb down one side of my body, which was pretty frightening,' she says. 'I ended up at this little hospital in Kathmandu, which looked more like a dusty wool shed. It was run by young American volunteer doctors and they thought I'd had a heart attack.' Terrified, Megan tried to fly home, but in those days the Nepalese travel agents didn't speak English well enough to change airline tickets, so she flew on to Greece before eventually returning to New Zealand.

When she reached the safety of her parents' property, Megan was taken to her local doctor for a thorough examination and diagnosis. 'The GP found nothing wrong with my heart whatsoever,' she recalls. 'He believed I had suffered from some sort of tropical disease that had affected my central nervous system.'

Back in New Zealand, Megan recovered quickly. She returned to her job at the bank, and throughout her twenties became quite career-minded. Even her beloved horseriding took a back seat for a while, though she continued coaching at the local pony club. She met Graeme, an insurance broker who was also a musician in a rock band. They got married, but soon after the wedding Megan suffered her second health event.

'I was 28 at the time and I was diagnosed with chronic fatigue,' she says. 'It came on immediately after the wedding and the doctors put it down to stress. There had also been horrendous floods in Gisborne, so it was a stressful time at work and in the community generally.'

Megan needed three months off work to recover, and it was a year before she was back to full strength. During her recovery she acquired a horse of her own again. 'As part of my recovery from chronic fatigue I started walking regularly, and the walk took me past the house of one of my riding students,' she remembers. 'I walked past one day and saw her horse had a bandage on its leg.' Megan knew her student was away at university, and the girl's parents didn't know much about horses. She offered to help out. 'I really got involved with this horse and I ended up buying it from the family.'

Life continued to be full and busy, and in time Megan became a rural bank manager at her branch. Thanks to her newly acquired horse she also started getting involved in riding again.

Then, when Megan was 33, her mother died suddenly and unexpectedly in her sleep. The following year, her father was killed in a terrible accident. 'I don't know if that was the catalyst, but from that time riding really took over my life again,' she remembers.

Megan and her husband made a lifestyle change, moving to Cambridge, the horseriding capital of New Zealand. They bought an acreage, and Megan took a part-time job with the bank so that she could concentrate on riding. Her horse duties took up at least three hours of every day—feeding, cleaning and riding. On weekends it was even more. Keen on showjumping in the past, Megan now became interested solely in dressage—the display of horsecraft that relies on core strength and subtle weight shifts from the rider. She competed locally, and was successful enough to gain entry into the national Horse of the Year event. At this elite level the winners' ribbons came with prize money attached. Not huge riches, but enough to cover the increasing costs of her hobby, the horse float, vet bills and feed. This last item was of particular interest to Megan as she groomed her horses for competitions. 'When you put a horse in a stable you are in control of everything that he eats, and you understand the influence you can have on his health with food and supplements,' she says. 'Magnesium, for example, is really important for horses because of their sheer muscle mass.'

Megan took great interest in nutritional science as far as her horses were concerned. 'I controlled the exact number of hours they were put out to grass at different times of year, and I knew the nutritional value of everything.'

Meanwhile, her own diet was being totally neglected. And she was overweight. 'I wasn't doing much cooking at all—I don't have a passion for it. We had a freezer full of meat—quality beef and mutton—and we ate a lot of that,' she says. 'And there was plenty of dairy too, cheeses and far too many chocolate biscuits.'

Throughout this period Megan might have got round to having children, but an emergency hysterectomy when she was 40 put an end to that idea. Still, her biological clock hadn't been ticking particularly loudly, and she was more than happy to enjoy her many nieces and nephews.

Five years later, in July 2005, Megan was sitting on her horse one afternoon, training for a dressage competition. Her instructor Sarah was watching from nearby as Megan attempted to make the horse trot forwards slowly. 'The horse started delicately side-stepping instead, which is very clever, but was the wrong thing to do,' explains Megan. 'I couldn't imagine why he was doing that,' she adds. In fact, Megan was losing feeling in the soles of her feet; she could no longer tell how much pressure she was putting on the stirrups, and the horse was receiving the wrong signals. 'In dressage the horse responds to the tiniest changes in pressure from the rider. I just didn't realise what I was telling my horse to do,' she says.

Megan then noticed that she was starting to get pins and needles in both feet. At first she thought this was linked to a back injury, but as the weeks went on and it gradually worsened she decided to consult her GP. 'He sent me to a sports doctor, still thinking the symptoms were injury-related,' says Megan. 'At this stage I was getting numbness down my left arm as well, and into two of my fingers.'

By now it was November. The sports doctor ordered an MRI, which showed up twelve lesions: nine on her spine and three in her brain. This specialist was the one to give Megan the news that it looked like multiple sclerosis. Megan reacted with anger, though not for the typical reason. 'I remember being really cross that I was being branded with a disease that bore my initials,' she says. 'I am Megan Swan, so my initials were already MS, and now I was going to have MS as well.'

The diagnosis was later confirmed by lumbar puncture, and by the time she got to see a neurologist her condition had deteriorated considerably. Megan wondered whether her earlier health events might be linked to the disease, but her neurologist said not necessarily. 'He diagnosed me straight away with primary progressive MS,' says Megan. 'By February 2006 I had gone on to lose all feeling up to my midriff, and my symptoms were continuing to worsen. They had started the previous July and got progressively worse over that time.'

The neurologist prescribed a dose of intravenous steroids, but Megan reacted badly to the drugs and her MS symptoms escalated further. 'It really threw me off my feet. I was feeling profoundly bad with terrible migraines,' she recalls. 'I was collapsing if I spent more than half an hour upright, and my thyroid function and digestion had been destroyed.'

Megan was told she was not eligible for disease-modifying drugs because she was not having defined relapses. 'I was just progressing and it was really terrifying. I had horrendous pain in my right arm, and migraines like you wouldn't believe.'

At this point Megan enlisted the help of a naturopath, to help her navigate the sea of supplements in a scientific way. 'He turned out to be a gifted physician and helped me enormously,' she says.

Once the after-effects of the disastrous dose of steroids wore off, Megan was still left with some serious MS symptoms to contend with. 'My energy levels were very low and I had terrible balance,' she remembers. 'Plus I still had the numbness in most of my body. I could walk, but I couldn't feel my body.'

Dressage training was out of the question, but Megan still had her horses to look after. She managed to waddle out to the paddocks, thanks to an old-fashioned pram that had been converted into a food cart. 'It became my mobility scooter,' Megan laughs. 'I loaded it up with buckets of food and I pushed it over to the horses. I'd never have been able to walk there on my own.'

One day, Megan was putting a halter on her horse and the urge took her to actually climb up. 'My balance was dreadful, but I just thought well, bugger this, I'm going to get on.' There was no saddle, but Megan managed to get herself up and onto the horse's back. 'I vividly remember that I was starting to slip off, leaning to one side. The horse somehow knew he had to look after me and he put himself underneath me,' she says.

And so began a gradual return to strength. 'Just being around animals is therapeutic,' says Megan.

Two other forms of exercise also played a large role in her early rehabilitation. The sports doctor who had initially diagnosed MS recommended cycling, so Megan found an old exercise bike and set it up at her house. To begin with, she could only manage five minutes a day, due to weakness in her muscles. 'After a few months I managed to get that up to an hour a day,' she says. 'I also joined a Pilates class, which was excellent for my balance.'

Unable to work for the first part of 2006, in August Megan started going in to the bank for just one hour every other day. This was more as a social rehabilitation than a real return to the workforce. 'Everyone at the bank was amazing,' she says. 'I had unlimited sick leave and the most understanding boss. I used to go in and just stay round the back and make tea or count coins—whatever I felt able to do,' she explains.

Her family too had rallied round to give her much-needed support. 'My sisters played a huge part in me staying sane throughout that time,' says Megan gratefully.

Her dressage coach Sarah, who was also a great friend, stayed in regular contact too. One day she appeared at the house with a copy of Professor George Jelinek's first book, *Taking Control of Multiple Sclerosis,* in her hands. Fascinated, Megan stayed up all night reading it, and by morning she was confused about what to make of the recommendations. She decided to get some advice from a local MS support lady, someone she'd met while in hospital who happened to share her interest in horses. Megan waited impatiently until 8.30a.m. and phoned this lady as soon as her office opened. 'I told her I had been given a book and I didn't know whether to throw it in the bin or live by it,' she recalls. 'She told me to live by it, and that's exactly what I did.'

At that stage Megan had not yet had breakfast. Nor was there much food in the house, except a freezer full of meat and a cupboard full of chocolate biscuits. Neither of those things were suitable for a low saturated-fat, wholefood, plant-based diet. 'I think I had toast and jam for breakfast, with no butter, and then I went shopping,' Megan says.

From that moment, Megan cut all meat and dairy out of her diet. Her expertise with horses meant that she understood the link between health and nutrition, but she adopted a rather harsh view of her situation. 'I really picked up on the diet, but not the mindset that needed to go with it,' she admits. 'In the early days I looked at the diet as a way of punishing my body for being ill. I thought yes, I'll beat this thing.'

In time she came to love the change in eating habits, but for quite a while the new regime was a struggle. 'I really wasn't much of a cook. In fact it was my husband Graeme who continued to do all the cooking at our house,' Megan says. 'He wasn't interested in following the diet himself, though he was happy for me to do it.'

Cutting out saturated fat was straightforward, but creating healthy food options was a real challenge. 'I ate a lot of bread,' Megan confesses.

Finding many of the recommendations quite difficult to incorporate into her life, Megan was tempted to consolidate what she had learned at a retreat. Her close friend and dressage coach Sarah offered to go with her. 'She really felt I needed a support person on board, and she thought there would be benefits for her own health as well.' By the time of the retreat in October 2006, Megan was still feeling quite low physically. She was weak, fainting occasionally, and extremely tired.

Over the course of the week, however, Megan started taking a serious look at her own life, coming to realise that she was in charge of her own destiny. 'I remember one session where we were encouraged to talk about the reasons why we had MS,' she says. 'Most people could pinpoint an exact event that triggered the disease.' Megan became rather self-conscious as she realised that she could identify no clear catalyst for what had happened to her. As the week went on, however, she started to see her past unravel.

'I began to think about my life and the way I had always dealt with stress. My attitude through everything that had ever happened to me was to put a brave face on things,' she recalls. 'I think that was a training that came from my parents, and I started to think it could have been my downfall.' Megan realised she had spent her life working very hard at achieving what other people thought she should achieve. 'I became a bank manager because that's what my father wanted. He was the real drive behind my career at the bank,' she says. 'I continued living my life as it was expected, rather than what I actually wanted. In the end MS exposed me,' she admits.

Megan felt that an accumulation of stress over many years finally became too much for her body to cope with. 'My way of dealing with things was doing the duck—staying calm on the surface, but going like hell underneath,' she remembers. This was accentuated by her training at the bank: the idea that you put on your lipstick, suit and smile, and that's your persona for the day. 'I really took that training on board, and when I rocked up for work I had the look and the attitude,' she says. 'I think I took it into other parts of my life as well.'

Megan's views started to shift during the retreat, not only in the way she saw herself, but also in how she approached her healing. 'My whole attitude changed. Instead of beating myself up over the diet,

I saw that I was rewarding myself with fantastic food.' She came away with a real conviction to change her life. 'I saw that the brave face wasn't getting me anywhere; I decided to be much more true to myself.'

For about a year she tried to do that from within her marriage. 'I thought I could survive that way,' she reflects.

But beginning to assess the energy that she both gained and lost from different situations, it became clear she needed to be on her own. 'I knew jolly well that even though some people meant well, they were still stripping me of energy,' she says. 'I made a decision to hang out with the people who lifted me up, and avoid the ones who sucked the energy out of me.' Unfortunately, Megan found that the main person who stripped her of energy was the one she lived with.

'I came to a decision that I needed to live on my own. Physically I was much better by then, and I was totally confident that I had found the answer to MS,' she explains. 'Spiritually I was in touch with my inner angels and I felt there was support for me there.'

Feeling that it was the most selfish decision she had ever made, Megan left her husband Graeme in February 2008. They later divorced.

Living alone, with no-one to answer to but herself, Megan began putting into practice some of the lessons she had learned at the retreat. For someone who just two years earlier had been diagnosed with primary progressive MS, her physical recovery was remarkable.

Most of her sensory issues had receded, leaving just a little numbness in her feet and legs. Her balance was not quite good enough to return to competitive horseriding, but she enjoyed brisk walking instead, clocking up many miles in the countryside around her new home. She had also returned to her part-time job at the bank, being careful to stay true to her own self when she put on the lipstick and uniform.

In 2009, keen to look deeper into the spiritual side of healing, Megan attended another retreat, this time with her sister Judy. 'It was absolutely as beneficial as the first, but in a totally different way,' she says. 'I learned more about myself, about my strengths and weaknesses, and I saw that I was setting a path forward for the future.'

That path, Megan fully expected, would see her happily settled in her new home near Lake Karapiro, surrounded by family and friends, living an active life. Alone.

In 2010, Megan felt so well physically she was jumping out of her skin. 'I really couldn't contain myself, I was just so fit,' she laughs. 'Being so well all the time and having so much energy, I used to go power walking for five kilometres (three miles) every day, but I really wanted to do more.'

Living by a lake, Megan became interested in kayaking. However, now aged 50, she was finding that many of her friends were busy with grandchildren and didn't have time for a new adventurous hobby. Arriving at her local salon for a haircut one afternoon,

Megan was greeted with the usual question, 'How's your love life?' from her hairdresser. 'Oh, I'm not interested in that,' she replied, 'but do you know anyone who wants to go kayaking?'

The lady in the chair next to her leaned across with a smile. 'I know someone you should meet,' she said. 'I know a guy who'd be just right for you.' Again Megan protested, saying she was looking for a kayaking partner, not a relationship. 'That's okay,' the lady replied, 'I think he'd enjoy kayaking too.'

Becoming slightly more interested at this point, Megan idly asked for some details. 'Well, his name's Graeme and he works in insurance,' came the reply. Megan immediately thought of her ex-husband. 'Absolutely not,' she laughed quickly, 'I don't need another Graeme who works in insurance!' Nevertheless, Megan took the phone number when it was offered.

Rather than returning to her home by the lake after her haircut, Megan went back to her friend's dog-boarding kennels. She was minding the place for two weeks while her friend was on holiday, but being confined to the property day after day was adding to her boredom and frustration. 'I thought if I don't have something to look forward to I'll go completely mad,' she says. 'So I rang the phone number I'd been given and arranged to meet this Graeme I'd been told about.'

Five weeks and five meetings later, Megan and the new Graeme were getting on really well, though they still hadn't been kayaking. 'At our age and stage we realised we'd need to work out fairly quickly if we were going to make it as a couple,' says Megan. 'Even though I hadn't been looking for romance at all, I did feel confident about entering a relationship. I no longer felt like a victim of MS and I believed I had great health to look forward to,' she muses.

That was lucky, because Graeme number two was in the process of finalising an adventure that would test the fitness of most 50-year-olds, let alone one with multiple sclerosis. A keen off-road four-wheel-driver, Graeme was organising a twelvemonth trip round Australia, camping on the roof of his truck, following the roughest tracks through the outback as far from civilisation as possible. Wardrobe space would be squeezed in between the chainsaw and the recovery gear, showers would be behind a tree, dinners would be cooked in a camp oven. And he wanted Megan to go with him. She jumped at the chance, though she was a little worried about the heat. 'I had read that people with MS often struggle in the heat, and we were going to be crossing several deserts,' she explains, 'so I bought a chiller vest and kept it at the ready in case I needed it.'

She never needed it. The year-long trip was challenging in many ways—physically tiring as she lived out of the back of the truck, exhausting as she pushed her body to the limit. But in all that time Megan's health never faltered, and in fact continued to improve.

Megan has two particularly triumphant memories from the trip, of physical feats she had never expected to be able to accomplish. The first was at Karijini National Park in Western Australia, when she and Graeme had gone on a particularly difficult canyon walk. The trip to Karijini had been an adventure in itself, the truck navigating some really rough tracks with vertical drop-offs. Megan often elected to hike rather than risk the extreme climbs and descents in the vehicle. At night they camped by clear pools and steep cliffs, and they went for days without seeing another person. Arriving at Karijini, Graeme and Megan hiked through deep gorges filled with stunning waterfalls and dramatic rock formations. The walks were graded from one to five, with five being the most difficult. 'Nearly all the walks we did were level five,' says Megan. 'They were very demanding and involved clambering across narrow ledges and wading through icy-cold water. At the end, to get out of the canyon we had to climb up the vertical rock face using a very long ladder,' she recalls.

A few weeks later the pair made their way across to Exmouth, where Ningaloo Reef gave Megan the chance to fulfil one of her lifetime ambitions. 'I had always dreamed of putting on a mask and fins and going snorkelling,' she says. She and Graeme joined a guided sea-kayaking tour and set out to explore the reef. 'We paddled for about an hour and a half in our tandem kayak and reached the reef, which was absolutely beautiful,' Megan remembers. 'I'm not a great swimmer, so snorkelling was a challenge, but I had the most amazing time. There was fabulous coral, sharks sleeping underneath rocks. And turtles,' she adds. 'I was really happy that I could keep up with these large turtles.'

The day had been just about perfect. But as they were about to return to the mainland a strong sea breeze blew up, making paddling very hard work. 'The other couples on the trip were all a lot younger than us, and the Indian Ocean was starting to get rather large waves on it,' Megan says. 'It was a long and tiring trip back, but we just kept paddling, kept helping each other, and eventually we made it to land,' says Megan. 'That trip was way more than I'd bargained for, but it was a great achievement. And I finally got the chance to go kayaking as well,' she laughs.

The Australian off-road adventure was so successful that Megan has built travel into her new lifestyle. For eight months of the year she lives out of a suitcase—though perhaps that is rather a grand word for it—while the other four are spent with family and friends back in New Zealand. Her health is almost perfect.

Almost. There was one event that threatened to derail her amazing recovery from MS, but fear soon turned to celebration. 'I had been home for a family wedding in March 2012, and right afterwards I started getting tingling in my feet like before,' Megan says. 'Then it spread up my legs and body—I was really quite concerned.' Megan took a low dose of steroids, which this time did not react badly with her body, and the disturbing symptoms soon faded. But it left her with a question: what had MS been doing to her brain and spinal cord for the past six years? Had the disease been silently progressing while she'd been off adventuring in blissful ignorance?

Megan decided to have an MRI to find out. 'I'm so glad I did,' she says. 'When I went back for the results I was told that there was absolutely no evidence of new lesions over the past six years. And the old lesions on my brain and spine were all disappearing, becoming more diffuse and faded,' she adds happily.

Megan was overjoyed. She returned to her life of adventure with Graeme, confident that she is truly overcoming multiple sclerosis. 'My expectations for the future are good health and good travel,' she says. 'I can't ask for more than that.'

10

A MODEL OF HEALTH

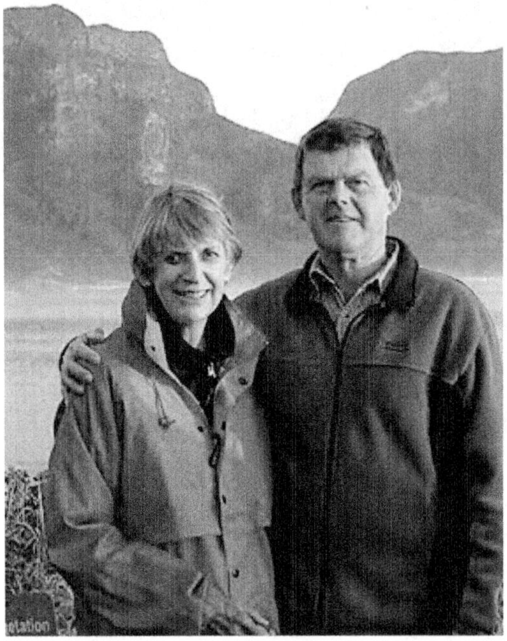

PHIL HASSELL

Once a week, in the quiet coastal town of Point Lonsdale in south-eastern Australia, a group of retirees get together. To meditate. It makes an interesting change from the charity work and the golf course, the walks along the beach and the time spent with the grandkids.

Former businessman Phil Hassell has been leading these sessions for the past three years, spurred on by requests from his friends. He arrives at the hall early each Wednesday evening, arranges the chairs in a welcoming circle, and waits quietly for everyone to arrive. Phil is now 67 and he's been meditating for nearly half his life. Since long before he was diagnosed with multiple sclerosis.

In fact it was way back in 1983 when, as a highly stressed sales executive, he was handed a book by a colleague who sensed it might be helpful. Out of interest and politeness Phil took the copy of *The Plus Factor: A guide to positive living* by Dr Harry Stanton, and started working his way through it. To begin with it didn't make much of an impression. 'I thought it was complete hogwash,' he admits. Halfway through the book, however, he tried out a meditation technique and it worked. The exercise involved building an imaginary stack of bricks in his mind from one to ten, then starting again. 'By the time I'd done that for 20 minutes I'd switched off from all my worries.'

Phil Hassell hadn't always had so much stress in his life. He grew up in country Victoria with his mum, older sister and two brothers. The family was very poor, but Phil didn't realise that at the time. They lived in a small weatherboard house, grew vegetables and kept a few animals. 'We had two sets of clothes, one for during the week and one for Sundays,' he says. Years later, at a school reunion, childhood friends told Phil they hadn't liked going to his house because there was never anything to eat. 'That's when I realised how poor we'd been,' he recalls. Still, his days were spent very happily roaming the countryside with his older brother; it was a gold-mining area so there were plenty of tunnels and shafts to explore. When evening approached Phil would return to the little house with its kerosene lanterns, wood stove and rainwater tanks. 'There was no power and nothing much to keep us inside the house so we spent all our time outdoors. We had a cow that we helped to milk, and a few chickens. Mum looked after the vegie patch and us kids were free to go where we wanted.'

When he reached school age, Phil walked the couple of kilometres to the small school with his siblings. By the time he reached high school the family had moved into Castlemaine, a bigger town of around 7500 people. After school he and his brothers would sometimes ride billy carts down the main street until they were chased off. Then they'd find a steep hill to ride them down instead. 'We used to live a bit dangerously,' says Phil. 'But it was nothing sinister, just boy mischief.'

When he was fifteen he started working a paper round to earn himself some money. 'I used to get up at 4.30a.m. and meet the train, sort papers, and then do my deliveries, and that's how I earned all my pocket money.' Understanding the value of the dollar, Phil turned out to be a hard worker and a very good saver. 'I'd set a goal and just go for it,' he remembers. 'I bought a new pushbike and a transistor radio, which were big things back then.' He even saved up and bought his first car, a green Austin A40, though he could rarely afford petrol. Luckily there were always plenty of mates around who could chip in.

By that time Phil was studying at technical college. 'I'd become quite unhappy at high school because maths was the only thing I was really good at, but they wanted me to study things like French and biology,' he recalls. 'So I went to the tech and I really blossomed.' Nevertheless, after just two years Phil was on the move again. 'I was quite unsettled, and because I had failed one subject I needed to repeat it the next year. I really didn't know what I wanted from life and I started looking around for jobs and ended up joining the RAAF [Royal Australian Air Force],' he explains.

Phil believes that was the making of him. 'It turned a boy into a man,' he says. New recruit Phil Hassell was a determined and hard-working young man who quickly became ambitious in his career. Over the space of twelve years he moved through the ranks in minimum time, gaining promotion to aircraftsman, leading aircraftsman, corporal and sergeant. Then he hit a brick wall. 'I was going for a commission to become an officer, but there was a change of government and they stopped allowing commissions from the ranks,' he says. Phil worked out that he would have to wait another eight years for his next promotion to flight sergeant. 'I wasn't prepared to wait that long, so I stayed until my signed term was up and then I got out.'

By that time he was 30 years old. He was also married with two young boys, the youngest just four months old when he left the forces. He had met his schoolteacher wife Judy during a posting to Malaysia some years earlier, and they had married on New Year's Eve in 1971. Always striving to better himself, Phil had also begun studying accountancy at that time, a part-time correspondence course which still had a short while to completion.

Phil, Judy and the kids moved from Melbourne to Woodend, a small, rural community at the base of Mount Macedon. Here they'd built a house on four acres (one and a half hectares). 'I like to have a bit of space around me, and it was enough land to grow all our own vegetables and run a few sheep,' he says. Phil got a job as a technical sales representative with a company he'd dealt with during his years in the military. Still very ambitious and with a tendency to perfectionism, he developed a successful career selling non-destructive testing equipment—ultrasonics, radiographics and electromagnetic equipment. It was a specialised field and after six years he'd become known for his expertise; Phil was head-hunted by another company and found himself leading a technical operation covering the whole of Australia.

Already fully committed in his work and family life, he also took on a large amount of community work. First it was the rural fire brigade, which he'd joined as soon as he left the airforce. Then when Woodend formed its own State Emergency Service (SES) branch in the town, Phil became a founding member. Soon he was an integral part of the organisation. 'Because of my airforce background I was made the first communication officer,' he says. 'Then I became the training officer, which covered just about everything, and I also became the deputy controller of the SES.' It was a lot of work on top of a busy job and family, but Phil enjoyed the extra challenge and always strove to do his best. 'There was training every week and often on weekends as well. Then I'd be called out to help with motor accidents and other disasters,' he adds.

The night of 16 February 1983 was the biggest disaster of them all. After ten months of drought, and with summer temperatures soaring and strong northerly winds ahead of a predicted westerly wind change, the whole community was on high alert. 'The fires were coming through and I was going on duty at midnight,' Phil remembers. 'I went to bed at 9p.m. and asked Judy to wake me if there was a wind change.' Five minutes later he got the call.

'The wind had stopped, and I knew the change was coming,' he says. Their own car was packed ready for Judy to drive the kids to safety, while Phil stayed to complete the fire-proofing of their home before starting his SES duties. That night, in what became known as the Ash Wednesday fires, seven local people lost their lives, and hundreds lost their homes.

'I was in charge of the evacuation centre in Woodend,' Phil remembers. 'We'd done all we could for our own house, set the soaker hose going on the roof with the downpipes blocked, and covered all the windows and doors.' The family home was saved, but there was a lot of damage. 'We lost sheds, a car, fences and walls, and 32 windows were broken,' Phil remembers. 'Embers got inside the house and burned through the carpet and lounge suite, and through papers from a meeting we'd had the night before—but luckily a fire didn't take off,' he says. It was a terrifying time.

And the very next day, in an unrelated quirk of fate, Phil's mother died of cancer.

Believing as he does that MS relapses are closely linked to stress, Phil might have expected the illness to have surfaced at exactly that point in his life. But it didn't—not for another fifteen years, in fact. The events of 1983 did, however, affect his health in other ways. 'By the end of that year I was pretty sick from stress. I was also working really hard, and every time it came to the weekend and I tried to relax I'd be violently ill with massive migraines and vomiting,' he says.

Phil's doctor ordered him off work for six weeks, but he only took three. 'I was trying to live up to everything I'd learned in management, and I was basically working 24 hours a day,' he confesses. 'I'd done a priority management course, which taught me to work to a very tight schedule all the time. I would read reports in the afternoon, let my subconscious work on it at night, make decisions in the morning. It was relentless.'

It was then that he first discovered meditation—that simple exercise of putting one imaginary brick on top of another, over and over again. 'I was really taken with it, but it was another few years before I started practising it in earnest,' he admits. By then Phil was working as an accountant, using the skills he'd learned on the correspondence course. 'I didn't tell the company about any of my technical skills, but the manager could see that I had more to offer, so I ended up taking on more responsibility anyway,' he says. Years later, back in technical sales and managing business in the southern part of Australia, Phil would close his eyes and meditate for 20–30 minutes every lunchtime. His staff used to joke about it, saying one day they would see him floating above the window. But he knew that without that breathing space he was unable to get through the day. Outside of work Phil gave away his SES duties, only to replace them with Rotary. Still, life was manageable. The boys grew up, left home, went to university. Phil and Judy moved back to Melbourne, and in 1998 Phil started his own business, again in technical sales. And that's when MS appeared.

In the beginning it was hard to pin down any actual symptoms, but there was an underlying malaise that seemed to be getting worse. He'd been complaining of tiredness for years, but now he started to make more frequent visits to his GP, looking for answers. 'My doctor told me I was working too hard, which was quite true,' Phil admits.

The fatigue wouldn't lift, however, and in March 2001, during a trip to Malaysia, he went for a run through the streets of Kuala Lumpur and struggled to finish it. That was very unusual, and although he was tempted to put it down to age—by then he was 55—it definitely worried him. Phil was a strong athlete who had been running for years, and he'd already started to notice that his times were getting slower. 'I could always run 3.2 kilometres (two miles) in around 11 minutes, then all of a sudden my time blew out to 14 minutes,' he says. For most people that might still seem a very respectable time, but Phil was concerned at such a sudden loss of strength and stamina. While in the airforce he'd competed professionally at long-distance running, and won the military services championships at 1500 metres and 5000 metres three years in a row. He'd kept up his fitness ever since, making running just one more item that he fitted into his busy schedule.

Returning home from Malaysia, it wasn't long before he noticed some numbness, first in his left foot and thigh, then travelling up into his torso. By June there was numbness in his arms and fingers as well, and he could feel a tight band of pressure around his lower chest. 'My left hip was in such jabbing pain that I was finding it difficult to walk,' he remembers. This time, when Phil turned up at his doctor's surgery looking for answers, his GP thought he'd had some sort of a stroke. That possibility was ruled out, but while waiting to see a neurologist the symptoms kept mounting. Phil started having trouble using the computer keyboard, and although his arm numbness receded during July, he experienced hot and cold feelings throughout his body, continuous lethargy and weakness. He carried on working though; a lifetime's habit was a hard one to break.

Finally, in November, his scheduled neurology appointment arrived. Phil was completely baffled by the growing list of symptoms, but he never considered MS might be to blame. 'I didn't have a clue what was wrong with me,' he admits. 'To begin with I'd thought the numbness and tingling might have been due to a pinched nerve from running.' Phil was shocked to discover that he had around six lesions in his lower neck and middle spine area, and several in his brain; two MRIs and a lumbar puncture made the diagnosis of relapsing-remitting MS conclusive.

'When I was diagnosed I was actually quite relieved, because I had something I could put a handle on; I knew what it was and I could do something about it,' he explains. 'That was my reaction—I didn't fall in a heap mentally.' Physically though, it was a different story. For the whole of the following year Phil continued to experience numbness, as well as dizziness and fatigue. He started losing his balance more often, and he realised that his cognitive skills were beginning to suffer. 'I couldn't concentrate for long periods of time,' he remembers. Phil was still working hard, running his own sales business, but he did start to make more time for holidays. When he was able to relax, he found that his symptoms eased slightly.

Throughout this period of early diagnosis Phil was not taking any medication. He was, however, put in touch with an MS nurse, who recommended Professor George Jelinek's lifestyle approach for managing the disease. Meditation was already an active part of his life, and exercise had featured highly for years. Diet, however, was something he had never really considered. He started assessing the food he was eating, but it wasn't until he returned from an MS retreat in 2003 that he actually began to make some changes. And even then, he wasn't 100 per cent committed to the program. Phil removed all meat and dairy from his diet, but he continued eating some processed foods. 'I'd have fish and chips when we went out, and I wasn't strict about the oils,' he admits. 'In my mind I thought so long as I kept saturated fat down I'd be okay.'

And in a way, he was okay. For the next few years Phil felt that his MS symptoms were controlled, but not necessarily reduced. He was able to continue running in the mornings, though not as strongly as he had before diagnosis. He kept on operating his business, though it was sometimes a struggle. And from time to time distressing symptoms would occur and interrupt his life, though they were never quite as debilitating as they had been when he was first diagnosed.

'Around the middle of 2004 my right arm started to get a bit shaky,' he says. 'I couldn't lift a cup of tea towards my mouth without wobbling it, and for a while I had difficulty controlling a pen to write.' He also experienced Lhermitte's sign, the neurological symptom where lowering the head leads to altered sensation in different parts of the body. In Phil's case his thighs and lower back were affected.

In 2005 Phil's neurologist was concerned at his deterioration, so Phil agreed to start taking Copaxone. Soon afterwards, a holiday on Lord Howe Island demonstrated just how much MS was affecting his health. 'I had bought a sport seat, which is a walking stick with three legs that you can also sit down on. I had to use that pretty much all the time,' he remembers. The island is known for its volcanic hills, some of which rise quite steeply from sea level. Phil struggled to navigate these, and the effort of walking knocked him about for a long time afterwards. 'There was one hill behind the lodge we were staying at, and it was not particularly high and was quite a gentle climb to the top,' he says. 'I managed to do it with my stick, but when I got back I was very tired and I was throwing my foot all the time.' The next day fatigue descended. 'We were walking along a flat road into the town area and I really struggled that particular day,' he remembers. 'It felt like there was no power in my right leg; I had a lot of trouble getting around on that trip.'

Back home Phil found that he only had energy for daytime activities, which still included work, but by the evenings he was spent. 'I used to sit inside the house—I really didn't go out much at night-time,' he says. Garden tasks were also getting a bit too much for him, so Judy had taken over the job of mowing the grass. 'It would just make me so tired if I tried to do it,' Phil recalls.

In 2006 Phil was told he had spasticity in his right leg, and was prescribed Baclofen to relieve it. 'I was getting quite intense pain in my right leg and buttock at night,' he says. The pain reduced, and he was able to exercise more strongly again. He gave up running, but turned to bike-riding instead. He also took up stretching and yoga, which seemed beneficial.

From the outside it looked as if Phil was doing all he could to take control of his health. He meditated every day, exercised nearly every day, had removed meat and dairy from his diet, and took Copaxone. Nevertheless his MS symptoms continued to trouble him. Then two more very important changes occurred. Firstly, Phil sold his business and retired. 'It was a mixture of being the right time to sell, and the fact that MS was making it so difficult,' he says. This instantly removed a huge amount of stress from his life. With time and energy freed up for other things, Phil and Judy booked into a follow-up MS retreat in July 2007, to immerse themselves in the lifestyle recommendations once more. And that's when the real recovery began.

'I realised I hadn't been doing things quite right—I just hadn't been rigorous enough,' Phil explains. 'I removed all processed food from my diet, bought organic whenever possible, stopped eating things that had been fried, and was specific in using only cold pressed virgin olive oil.' He also started supplementing with both flaxseed oil and vitamin D, which he had never done before. 'I was given a UV meter by a friend from the retreat, and I set it up in the garden. I monitored my time in the sun quite closely and boosted my vitamin D levels.'

It was like starting all over again for Phil, and after just a few months of tightening up on his lifestyle he found that his energy, strength and stamina had noticeably improved. He started going out to work in the garden most days. Not mowing yet, but digging, planting, raking and clearing. Some days he struggled to keep going, but mostly he was able to do quite lengthy physical work. 'I realised I was stronger than I had been the previous year,' he says.

There were improvements on the golf course too. Not with his swing or putting, but with his stamina in walking round all eighteen holes. In December 2007 he played a full round of golf without using a buggy, and only tired on the last three or four holes. Just before Christmas that year he walked briskly along a 2.5 kilometre (one and a half mile) beach path. It was a once-familiar track that he'd stopped using in recent years. He needed to rest on the way back, but he was delighted to find that his body still felt strong at the finish.

Phil's rigorous lifestyle regime continued, and partway through the following year he took up running again. After several months he found that his right leg was getting stronger, which in turn enabled him to exercise more. In February 2009 he decided to take part in the MS Melbourne Cycle event, a 40 kilometre (25 mile) ride with a group of colleagues. Judy entered too, and for the first 22 kilometres (thirteen and a half miles) Phil stuck at her pace. Then, with half the distance still to go, he rode as fast as he could to the finish. 'I was definitely tired when I cycled up that last hill and I had to change into a low gear,' he says. 'But I only finished a few minutes behind the other team members.'

By now Phil was becoming more confident of his health. He knew he was in much better shape than he had been two years earlier. And the improvements continued. Now able to run along the beach path, he soon found he could run up and down the steps from the path, completing eight repetitions. He also put in some hard bike rides, covering 10 kilometres (six miles) in just 27 minutes.

But then disaster struck. Phil and Judy were driving through the countryside near Geelong one afternoon when they were involved in a horrific car accident. They were lucky to survive; emergency workers said the car they were driving, a Mercedes, was what saved them. However, the crash was still extremely traumatic. Judy spent eight weeks in hospital, and Phil ten days. But his right leg, still weak from eight years of MS, was badly smashed at the foot. Their children, by then married with kids of their own, came to Phil's hospital bedside. 'When the doctors were explaining my injuries, they mentioned that I would be left with a limp in my right leg,' Phil says. His children listened before telling the doctors with a chuckle, 'He's already got one!' That was quite true, as Phil had been walking with a pronounced limp for about five years.

The car accident brought great support from Phil's social circle, and it served to highlight his chosen lifestyle to his friends. 'When I came out of hospital the members of Probus drew up two rosters,' he remembers. 'One was for people to drive me to visit Judy, who was still on the ward, and the other was to provide a meal for me every day.' Phil's eating habits became the talk of the town. 'People really went to a lot of trouble to feed me the right stuff, and I had some wonderful meals,' he remembers gratefully. Many members of the community were aware of Phil's other lifestyle changes too, and started to take more of an interest. 'People began asking me about meditation; they were interested in it and wanted help getting started,' he recalls. 'After the accident, both Judy and I decided that since our lives didn't end there, we must be around for a reason,' Phil says. He took the plunge and started a local meditation group. 'I think people see me as a role model. One couple have changed their diet and now meditate every day.'

Phil's physical rehabilitation from the car accident included strenuous running and weight resistance. He'd been told that he would be left with residual damage, but Phil decided otherwise. And he was proved right. As he recovered from his injuries and his strength returned, so his recovery from MS received another boost. 'I joined a weight-resistance training group and that really improved my strength,' he says. By 2011 Phil was running, mowing the grass, playing golf regularly, and enjoying quality time in the evenings without the burden of fatigue. His Lhermitte's sign had gone, and his longstanding limp had also disappeared. 'Friends on the golf course certainly commented on how well I was getting around, and I was able to keep up with the grandkids a lot better, having fun with them and playing football,' he muses. A few years earlier he would have been watching from the sidelines, unable to join in.

In September 2012, Phil returned to Lord Howe Island for another holiday. Again he and Judy travelled with a group of friends, hoping to enjoy the mountainous walks and the golf together. Seven years earlier Phil had tired easily and lagged behind the others. But this time it was different. He now had the energy and physical fitness to keep up with his friends, and some members of the group were even struggling to keep up with him. 'I used a couple of walking poles to help me on the rough ground, but there were no restrictions for me physically on that trip at all,' he says happily. 'I played eighteen holes of golf on a course that looked like it was made for mountain goats,' he laughs. 'On our first day we walked up one of the mountainous ridges with a pretty steep ascent,' he remembers. 'I was still fine in the afternoon after doing that, and the next day I was able to walk into town and enjoy everything with no problems.'

Like most people in their mid sixties, Phil does feel tired at the end of a long walk; it is the symptoms of MS he has managed to reverse, not the ageing process. But overall his health is astonishing. 'Really for the last two years I have had very few symptoms. If I play eighteen holes of golf then I need a rest at the end of it. But then so do all the guys I play with,' he says. 'I can walk that five kilometre (three mile) beach path, and I can complete ten repetitions up and down the steps. I guess the only noticeable thing would be that if I walk really hard for six kilometres (four miles) or so, I start throwing my foot at the end of it,' he explains. 'And some days I am a little more tired in the evenings.'

Phil believes that sticking 100 per cent to the diet and lifestyle recommendations is the reason for his current good health. 'When I realised that I wasn't quite doing everything I needed to do it really changed things,' he says. 'I became far more rigorous with the diet, exercise, meditation, flaxseed oil and vitamin D. I'm sure that is why I have just gradually improved over these last few years.'

Now confident of his health, Phil is delighted that he can look forward to the rest of his retirement. The golf, the garden, the walks, the time spent with the grandchildren. And, of course, being a role model for good health to his friends and community.

11

HARNESSING A REBELLIOUS STREAK

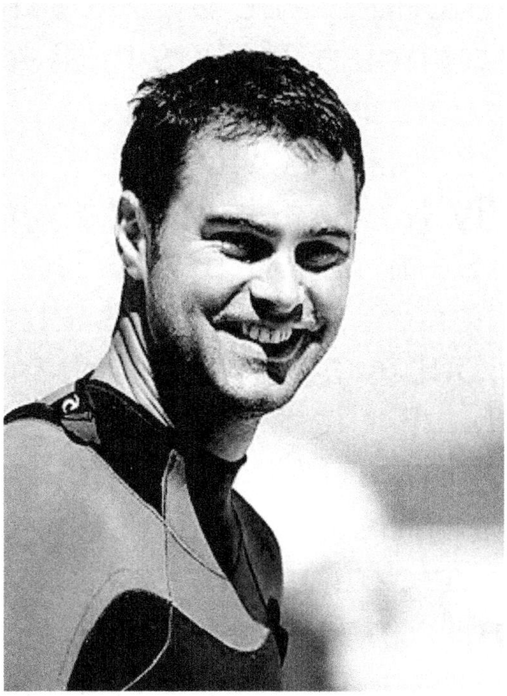

SAM GARTLAND

Sam Gartland has always had a rebellious streak. Long before he started training to become a doctor, he was causing minor mayhem for the teachers at his south-east London primary school. It was never anything serious or malicious, just Sam's rather individual slant on the world, fuelled by a sharp intelligence and big sense of humour. He was suspended from primary school once for letting off a stink bomb during a church assembly. At high school Sam continued to challenge authority for a few years, making moderately frequent visits to the principal's office. Then, when he was fifteen, his love of learning took over and he became serious about his studies. He still had plenty of time for fun, though, and by the time he was ready for university the choice of Manchester was made—for its nightlife as much as for its highly regarded medical curriculum.

'I had a really happy childhood—loads of fun and a great family,' Sam remembers. He was the middle one of three children, with sisters either side of him. 'I did get into trouble a bit, but I was pretty creative in my thinking back then.'

There was even a hint of rebellion in his choice to study medicine, as it was breaking away from his parents' artistic background. Sam's dad was a stage actor in London, running his own theatre company for a while, and his mum was a college English lecturer. 'My parents were very arty and I guess I wanted to do something different,' he muses. 'I was interested in the human body and I was keen on science. I thought medicine would give me an insight into people and how things work.'

Sam took a year off after leaving school, teaching English in Borneo for a while and travelling the world. Arriving in Manchester in 1993, his young mind was ready to take on the challenges of medicine, learning the science that would hopefully enable him to make a valuable contribution to healthcare one day. But his free, creative spirit soon crumpled under the onslaught of rote learning and formulaic science. 'Any commonsense was knocked out of me at a very early stage,' he admits. 'Even at high school when I was taking chemistry A level, all you had to do was regurgitate a lot of formulas and you got top grades,' he says. 'Manchester Medical School had developed a problem-based curriculum, which was an improvement, but at the end of the day we were still learning about purely pharmaceutical-based treatments or surgery.'

Still, Sam doesn't like to be too critical. After all, pharmaceuticals and surgery were the only options his lecturers had learned about too. And it took Sam a long time to open his eyes and mind to other possibilities as well—even when his own health depended on it.

Sam's university years passed smoothly enough. He was fairly hard-working, and he enjoyed the nightlife as well. Like many students he got a part-time job in a bar to earn extra cash, and for sport and exercise he took up Thai boxing. 'I used to train for eight hours a week. It was quite energetic, with lots of pounding, kicking and punching. It was run by Thai people, and at the end of each session we would do a 20-minute meditative breathing exercise.' That was Sam's first exposure to anything like meditation, and he found it helpful for calming the anxiety that had started to creep into his life. 'Unfortunately the meditation left my life before I got ill,' he says.

After six years of medical studies, including several internships at hospitals to gain practical experience, Sam was ready for the gruelling regime dished out to all new doctors. 'I remember working long hours and horrible shift patterns. As a junior doctor you are given a lot of responsibility when you are still very inexperienced, which can be quite stressful,' he explains.

He stayed in Manchester for a while, before moving down to London. Life was busy and outwardly successful, but not particularly happy. 'I was in a very fractious relationship, so my personal life wasn't great. And at work I was struggling to decide which area of medicine I really wanted to be in,' he recalls. The burden of his future career direction came to preoccupy him more and more as the months went on. 'I was really churning it over in my mind, never feeling satisfied,' he admits. 'I felt very mixed up inside and didn't really know what to do.'

When he was 27, Sam went to Australia to work at a Sydney hospital. Here at least he could indulge his passion for surfing and let some joy back into his life. But the Australian dollar wasn't strong enough to allow Sam to pay off his large student debt, so after just a year he reluctantly moved back to England.

The next few years saw him working as a hospital physician, a GP and an intensive care doctor. 'I was sort of driven in my job, but at the same time I didn't really know what I wanted to do and it caused me real angst,' he admits. 'In reality life was fantastic, but internally I had this thought process that drove me nuts.'

A hectic social life helped to push thoughts of his future into the background. Now living in Manchester again, Sam spent his free evenings at nightclubs with his medic friends. He no longer lived alone, having moved in with his new partner Lisette, but at that time he didn't feel especially settled. It was a fast-paced, high-energy existence that combined long working hours and study for further exams with a slightly crazy nightlife. 'My world was devoid of all spirituality,' he admits.

Around the time of his 31st birthday, Sam was working in intensive care. He had recently sat for the second part of his written exams for entry to the Royal College of Physicians. 'I knew my thinking had become foggy, so I wasn't surprised when I failed the exam by half a per cent,' he says.

There were other signs that Sam's mind and body were starting to fail, though it was tempting to put it down to the demands of medical life. 'Working shifts made it very hard to get enough sleep, and I knew I didn't feel good in myself,' he says. 'I was struggling to go into work, but I thought maybe that's just what happens when you turn 30—that you just can't push your body so hard anymore.'

In fact it was the start of Sam's first episode of multiple sclerosis and it wasn't long before the symptoms became much more obvious and disturbing. 'Towards the end of the year I noticed some numbness in my legs, but it wasn't there all the time,' he says. 'Then, at the start of 2008, it got a lot worse.' One Sunday morning Sam was on a ward round at the hospital when his emergency pager went off. Hearing the signal, he reacted instantly and tried to run to assist. 'My legs just wouldn't move. I was trying to make them run but they just wouldn't do it,' Sam recalls. Luckily the emergency crash call was cancelled, but as he resumed his ward round he told the consultant what had happened. 'I knew this was bad, and I told her I was really worried. Incredibly, she said I would have to see someone about it on Monday because we had a ward round to complete,' he says.

When Monday came around, Sam was giving a presentation at work. 'I totally lost it—I was falling asleep trying to give the talk, and my legs had gone numb just walking from the car park,' he remembers. Sam was sent for an MRI, but he was already well aware that his symptoms pointed to something serious.

'One of the doctors put my scans up next morning at the daily trauma meeting where they discuss cases,' says Sam. 'As soon as he had it up on the screen, he pulled it down again straight away. He'd obviously seen something, so he asked me to come to his room.' What the consultant had seen was a lesion in Sam's thoracic cord and a lesion in his brain, likely to be the start of MS. Sam was sent away to wait and see what might develop. He was given a course of steroids and he needed three months off work to recover. 'That was really weird because I had actually never had a break from work before,' he says. During that time the numbness in his legs subsided and the overwhelming fatigue lifted.

Around this time a physician friend, who also had MS, lent him Professor George Jelinek's first book. Sam read it and thought about making some changes, in a rather half-hearted way. 'I didn't actually know that I had MS yet,' he says. 'The book had piqued my interest but I hadn't taken it fully on board.'

Just before Sam returned to work he went kite-surfing for a week in the Mediterranean; his body felt strong again and some calmness had returned to his life. But neither of those feelings would last very long.

Sam went back to his job in the intensive care ward and within months he had a second relapse, which confirmed the MS diagnosis. This time his vision was affected with blurring in his right eye, and once again he was hit with crippling fatigue, numbness and weakness in his legs. He took a month off work and tried to return, but it soon became obvious that the workload was just too much for him. And if it was obvious to Sam, it was even more obvious to his senior doctors and consultants at the hospital. 'They made it quite clear to me that I would have to leave my job. I was told to take the next few months off and consider what I was going to do,' he recalls. 'I even received a text message suggesting I should take retirement due to ill health.'

Sam was forced to take another extended break from work. He spent his days alone in the house he shared with Lisette, with his mood and state of mind in a downward spiral. With many qualified doctors, consultants and even neurologists among his friends, he was not short of opinions on his distressing situation. 'I remember phoning one friend to tell him the diagnosis and he said, "Oh well, you're the right age for it." Other people from work just wouldn't look me in the eye when we met,' he remarks.

The prevailing medical view was that MS could be partially managed with disease-modifying drugs, but was nevertheless progressively disabling. Sam had first learned this as a medical student at university. 'I remember looking at this picture of a brain of someone with MS and thinking God, I really don't want to get that,' he says. 'Later when I did a neurology attachment as a junior doctor we diagnosed a young woman who'd developed MS. It was all very serious and hushed because there were no effective treatments, and we couldn't reassure her about the future,' he remembers.

Sam's years as a doctor had brought him into contact with many people with MS, and as a rule they had fared badly. It was the young men Sam remembered best. 'Manchester has a very high prevalence rate of MS—about one in 500. A lot of the men I saw seemed to deteriorate very rapidly.' Sam vividly recalls breaking into the house of one young man who had fallen out of his wheelchair. 'He had a urinary infection and needed to be taken to hospital. It wasn't a pretty sight.'

These rather grim images of life with MS were constantly playing on his mind. He had of course been offered a different view, but he was finding it hard to reconcile the suggested lifestyle options with his years of medical training. 'I'd read the evidence for diet and lifestyle and on one level I could see that it made sense,' says Sam. 'But at that time I saw MS as so powerful that when my body's immune system turned on itself I couldn't see what I could do to stop it. It was beyond my comprehension that changing the way I lived could actually reverse that,' he admits. Sam's thinking had become very rigid as a medical doctor. 'I thought surely if there was something in this then I would have been taught it. I was under a well-regarded MS specialist in Manchester, and when I mentioned it to him he just shrugged.'

So Sam continued with his typical northern English lifestyle. He was such a regular at the local kebab shop that he got special discounts, and the curry house where he ate twice a week had his photo in their 2008 calendar.

Previously plagued by thoughts about the future direction of his medical career, in 2008 it looked as if Sam wouldn't have a medical career at all. Continuing with his specialist training was futile, so he started applying for part-time GP positions for which he was already qualified. 'On a number of occasions I was at the point of taking a job,' he remembers. 'Then they would find out about my MS diagnosis and I would hear no more.'

Sam then experienced another flare-up of symptoms, and hit a real low point in his life. 'I'd lost my job and I couldn't find another one to go to. Physically I was in a mess, and my personal life was in trouble as well. I was becoming horrible to live with and my behaviour was putting a strain on my relationship with Lisette,' he admits.

Seeing how much Sam was struggling, his mum and dad stepped in and reminded him of the other options. 'They had been looking on The Gawler Foundation website and they told me it said the science was clear: that if you make these lifestyle changes you can halt the disease. I remember saying that was a big claim to make,' says Sam. 'At that time I still couldn't see it.'

It took a family trip to Granada to start to change Sam's mind, and things still had to get worse before they got better. His mum and dad were celebrating their wedding anniversary and, unusually for the Gartlands, they had organised a long weekend away together with all three children to mark the occasion.

By this time Sam's parents and his two sisters had read up on the lifestyle options for MS and were hopeful it could make a difference for Sam, if he was prepared to try. The restaurant table was beautifully set for the family's first meal of the holiday. Sam knew that all eyes were on him as he sat down to order. 'Everyone was looking at me wondering if I was going to choose an "appropriate" meal,' he says. 'The more I thought about it, the more I knew I would eat whatever the hell I wanted.' Everyone looked on in horror as Sam's voice rang out. 'I'd like the lamb,' he said firmly to the waiter. His mum erupted, the celebration was ruined, and Sam felt ostracised for the remainder of the weekend.

However, this harsh treatment did finally start to have an effect. By the end of the trip he had come round to the idea of booking into an MS retreat in Australia. Two things helped to change his mind. The first was the fact that George Jelinek was an emergency physician, and when Sam had worked in Sydney he'd been impressed by the pragmatic approach of the Australian emergency doctors. The other was that Sam's rebellious streak—his creative free-thinking mind—was starting to be rekindled.

Despite the difficulties in their relationship, Lisette chose to attend the retreat with Sam to support him and together they travelled to Australia in February 2009. It was six months since Sam had last worked as a doctor, and he desperately needed some good news. 'As soon as I walked into the retreat and saw

George Jelinek, I knew he had found an answer to MS,' says Sam. 'He just looked so well, so vibrant, and I knew that this solution was real.'

As Sam listened to the evidence about diet, vitamin D, exercise and meditation his conviction grew. He also realised that by embracing the changes he was choosing to value and look after himself. 'I felt like my whole being could let out a giant sigh and that I could finally let go,' he says. 'It changed everything for me.'

From a scientific and medical point of view, the evidence made sense to Sam. He remembered reading some research papers on vitamin D and MS when he was first studying medicine. He'd wondered at the time why no-one had followed up on this promising line of enquiry. Now his idle questioning turned to outrage and disbelief. He came to similar conclusions about the other aspects of the recovery program, and by the time he flew back to Manchester he was sure that a lifestyle approach could stabilise MS and reverse the symptoms he was still experiencing. 'At that time I was still getting numbness from the waist down, and fatigue was a big problem for me,' he says. He had started Copaxone injections a few months earlier, and decided to stay on the drug while he addressed his lifestyle.

Now convinced of the need to change, Sam had no difficulty altering his fast-food habit to a wholefood, plant-based diet plus seafood. 'A lot of people are quicker to catch on than me,' he admits. 'The first time I read the evidence I didn't really believe it, or perhaps I was in denial, but I wasn't able to make any changes. Once I truly believed this was going to work, changing my habits was quite easy,' he says. Lisette adopted all the dietary changes too. 'She was incredibly supportive, helping with meals and cooking healthy treats,' he adds.

Back in Manchester, Sam had his vitamin D level tested and found, not surprisingly, that he was quite deficient. 'I lived in a place with low sun exposure all year round, and I spent most of my time indoors,' he explains. He supplemented and quickly lifted his levels to above 150 nmol/L.

Having learned mindfulness meditation on the retreat, Sam found it incredibly helpful for calming the anxiety that was often present in his life. 'I got into a regular practice of meditation and I found it an excellent buffer from all the little things that come up. It was something I needed—a natural restorative process that improved my overall functioning.' Back home he felt mentally more able to cope with his diagnosis, and he consulted a psychologist who used mindfulness techniques to alter his thought patterns. 'She really built on what I had already learned. I was over-anxious and caught up in things, and this was the first time anyone had told me I had control over which thoughts to follow.'

Sam was finally successful in securing a job as a GP, though to begin with his hours were very limited to accommodate his symptoms. 'I worked for two days a week, with a big gap in between those days to give me the best possible chance to recover,' he says. 'It was a practice in a very rough part of the city, but I enjoyed the work.'

Six months after leaving the retreat, Sam noticed some real physical improvements to his health. His legs felt stronger and no longer went numb so often, and his energy levels had also increased. Sam returned to Thai boxing and later joined a soccer team. 'I played with a lot of radiologists, and as I continued to get better one of them asked if I was sure I'd been diagnosed correctly,' he remembers.

As Sam's body became stronger, he increased his working hours until eventually he was working full time again. Along the way he re-sat the second part of his physician exam, the one he had failed by half a per cent in 2007. 'When I went to take the exam they said that I could have extra time if I needed it because of MS. Physically I was okay, but my powers of concentration were not so good.' Sam decided not to ask for extra time, and he easily passed the exam. 'I could tell my cognition was improving again,' he adds.

Thankfully Sam's relationship survived the turmoil following diagnosis, and this also brought more stability into his life. For the first time Sam was feeling clearer about who he was and what he wanted to do with his life. The anxiety he'd been living with for so long was starting to fade. 'Getting MS allowed me to make all these changes, and I suddenly started to really enjoy life again,' he reflects. 'I had been completely self-obsessed and self-absorbed for a long time. Mentally this was my chance to rediscover who I was.'

It wasn't only Lisette who noticed the changes in him. 'My older sister commented to my mum one day that she was glad to have her little brother back again,' Sam says. 'I felt stronger and happier and clearer in my thinking than I ever had before. I know this sounds silly, because theoretically I was doing exactly what I wanted to do when I was diagnosed with MS,' he says. 'But MS gave me the right to relax.'

When Sam first became sick he felt strongly drawn to nature, and knew he felt better when he spent time outdoors. 'I realised that all I'd ever really wanted to do was go surfing.' In October 2010, he secured a contract to work as a GP in regional Australia, and both he and Lisette moved from Manchester to the central coast region of New South Wales. Here Sam finetuned his new lifestyle with plenty of exercise, sunshine, meditation and laughter. Over the months his health and strength continued to improve.

Keen to make the move permanent, Sam applied for Australian residency, but was refused on health grounds. 'They were worried I was going to cost the country thousands of dollars in medical expenses.' Unwilling to take no for an answer, Sam's rebellious spirit took over. 'It had been a pretty damning letter from the Australian government stating that I had a disabling condition that was only partially treatable with strong drugs,' he says. 'This didn't seem to reflect what I now knew about MS at all,' he adds.

Sam enlisted the help firstly of George Jelinek, who wrote a letter supporting Sam's good health and affirming that he expected him to remain well in the future. Next he called on the local surf lifesavers with whom he'd recently taken his bronze medallion. And lastly the captain of the local over-35s soccer team stated that Sam had played every game that season and made a very valuable contribution to the side. 'The government accepted my appeal and I was granted permanent residency,' Sam says happily.

The following year he and Lisette got married. In time they bought a house near the ocean, close enough for Sam to go surfing in the mornings before work. It had taken almost three years for his body and mind to completely recover from the spate of MS relapses, but by early 2012 he was feeling strong, calm and confident about the future.

Halfway through the year, the GP practice where Sam was working suggested he should consult a neurologist. They had sponsored Sam for residency and wanted to be sure that he was getting the best possible medical advice, and was linked to a specialist in case he ever needed one. 'I didn't really want to see a neurologist because I felt completely fine, but part of me wanted to show them how well I was after following the program,' he admits. So Sam went along and told his story of diet and lifestyle intervention followed by recovery. 'After my appointment I got a letter back requesting that I have an MRI scan,' he says. 'I was partly curious, because I knew of other people who had changed their lifestyle and then found that their scans improved.'

Arriving for the MRI, Sam immediately felt vulnerable again. 'Every now and then you have those anxious moments, and lying there inside the scanner I suddenly felt very small,' he admits. 'I started wondering if I was mad to imagine that I had got better. Perhaps it was all in my head? What would I do if my recovery turned out not to be real?'

It was a confronting moment, and Sam was in no hurry to go back and collect his results. Being a doctor, he opened up the envelope and held the scans up to the light when he got back to his house. 'I thought everything looked fine. There didn't seem to be any lesions there at all,' he remembers. Still, he knew he had to wait for the neurologist's verdict before coming to any real conclusions.

Work was busy and on the day of the follow-up appointment Sam was running very late. When he finally arrived, the neurologist had deliberately stayed behind in order to see him.

'He said he had some very good news for me. All the old lesions had gone and there was absolutely no evidence of MS on my scans whatsoever,' Sam laughs. 'In fact, the neurologist had trouble believing that I had ever had MS in the first place. He told me that I must have had two clinically isolated attacks,' he says.

Sam pointed out, quite rightly, that this was an oxymoron. One attack could be considered isolated, but two or more gives you the diagnosis of MS.

'It seemed beyond the neurologist's comprehension to accept that I might have recovered,' says Sam. 'His body language was very defensive; he sat with his legs crossed and his arms crossed, and told me that it couldn't have been MS.'

The neurologist also suggested that Sam could stop taking the Copaxone that he'd been injecting every day for the past three years. 'That was quite a challenging thing for me to consider, but I knew he was right when he said the drugs just aren't that good,' says Sam.

Just a few years earlier, Sam had just as much trouble believing that recovery from MS was possible. 'My robotic thinking was probably helpful in emergency situations, but it didn't allow me to see the real picture with MS,' he says. 'I held certain medical beliefs, and for a long time I thought that what happened to my body was totally out of my own control.'

Today Sam sees things very differently. He believes that circumstances led to MS being present in his life, and that his own actions are responsible for it now being absent. 'I was born in March, so my mum had low vitamin D exposure during pregnancy. Then I moved to northern England, which also has low sun exposure. My diet was typical Western—high fat, refined food—and I had a lot of anxiety in my life. I was working shifts, which we know increases the risk of MS, and I even had a genetic predisposition because a distant aunt had the disease,' reflects Sam. 'That reads like a complete recipe for MS. But when you reverse those environmental risk factors then you get better, and that isn't a surprise,' he says with a grin.

Now he is looking for ways to integrate his new understanding of medicine into his clinical practice. 'Ultimately there's no more important thing to do than help people understand that there are different ways of approaching things. People have to be given a choice,' he says. 'With many chronic diseases you can either carry on the way you are and gradually deteriorate over time, or you can radically change the way you live and feel completely better,' he explains.

He knows this view is unfashionable and somewhat outside the conventional medical paradigm, but that's okay. After all, Sam Gartland has always had a rebellious streak.

12

A BREATH OF HOPE

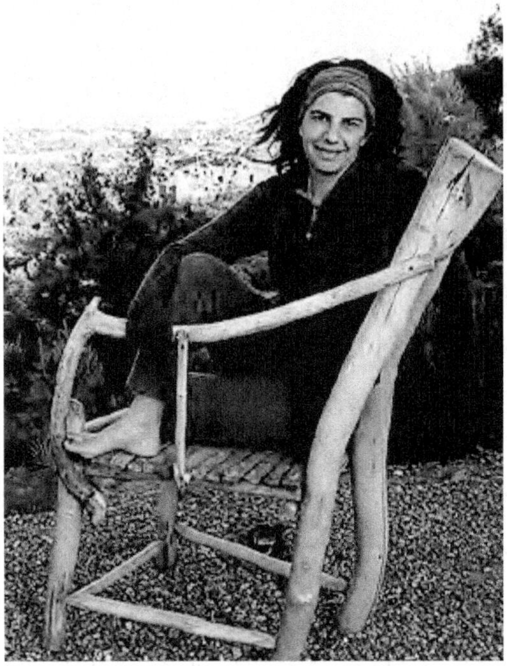

LINDA BLOOM

Linda Bloom grew up in a typical suburban house in Melbourne, Australia: a quiet street, a flat yard for playing, and a caravan round the side for family holidays. Linda's childhood would have been totally unremarkable except for two facts—her parents' cultural background and her mother's death from breast cancer when Linda was just six years old.

Her parents were Hungarian Jews who had survived the holocaust when most of the extended family were killed. The few who survived either emigrated to Israel, or remained in Hungary until 1956; when the revolution hit, they found themselves fighting for their lives once again. Linda had often heard the story of how her parents walked into a registry office in their snow boots to get married, fleeing Hungary the next day as refugees on a journey that would eventually bring them to Australia. Her grandma and a very few other relatives fled too, leaving Hungary with only the clothes on their backs, and finally ending up in Melbourne. With determination and extremely hard work they managed to make a good life for themselves, Linda's father working as an engineer, but with their history always close to the surface.

'They were tough cookies,' Linda remembers. 'I grew up listening to lots of stories about the harrowing decisions they had to make in order to survive.'

Those stories were mostly told by her grandma, who played a central role in Linda's life, moving into the family home to help look after Linda's family when her mother became sick. Those early years of childhood were difficult and Linda has few memories from that time, but she does recall her grandma being the rock on which everything depended, living in the house with them through her mother's illness, her death on 18 August 1980, and the period that followed. Her father was also a constant support for Linda and she looked up to him with love and admiration.

Two years after her mother died, Linda's father remarried, to a lady who loved Linda like her own child. Her new 'Mum' was a loving, caring, affectionate woman who shared Linda and her father's sense of humour and instantly became an important member of the family. Unfortunately, she also had health problems that were difficult for her and the family to navigate. From a young age, some family situations led to tensions in the house. With her sister already married and living her own life, Linda felt like it was her responsibility to try to resolve the difficulties at home and make everything okay.

'I became the peacemaker, which in retrospect I can see was not my role at all. It was my way of trying to take control of a situation that at times felt out of control—though it took me a very long time to realise that,' she says.

Over the years the young peacemaker grew into a confident, open-hearted, successful young woman. As a teenager she remained eager to please, perhaps satisfying others more than herself. Her generous nature may have made that easier to achieve, but while she was studying at university and partway through her psychology degree, a situation arose that prompted her to act differently for the first time.

Now aged 20, Linda had spent many years saving up to go travelling, sometimes working several part-time jobs simultaneously. By 1994 she had finally saved enough money to head to Europe. Postponing her studies for a year, she set off with a backpack, a friend and all her available funds to enjoy a well-earned taste of freedom and adventure. She did this with the support of her family, who knew she would be back the following year to continue her studies.

The year of travel was all she hoped it would be. Just prior to coming home, and leaving all her belongings at her uncle's house in Hungary, she booked a return flight to New York for a two-week trip.

'I just took a toothbrush and a T-shirt and very little else,' Linda remembers. 'I wasn't planning to be there for long.'

But as soon as she reached New York, she fell in love with the place and decided to stay.

'It was right at the end of my trip, so I'd pretty much run out of money by then and I was enrolled to go back to university for the following year. But I was just really sure and really determined that this was what I was going to do,' she explains. 'When I phoned Dad to tell him, it was a pretty traumatic conversation because I had always done what I was told, and this was the first time I'd really stood up for myself. My dad and I had always shared a close and loving relationship; I knew that if I needed him he'd be there for me no matter what,' Linda says. But this time it was different.

'He told me that if I stayed I would be on my own—he would not support me. It was very dramatic. But I'd made my decision and I felt like I really grew up at that moment, doing what I needed to do for me rather than for anybody else.'

Linda stayed in New York and it turned out to be the best year of her life. She had to work fourteen-hour days to make enough money to survive. She moved into an apartment with a friend, worked and played hard, and ultimately proved that she could survive on her own. 'That whole experience taught me to trust myself, and the rest would follow,' she says.

The year in New York was important for another reason, too: it was where Linda was introduced to meditation. Never having any particular spiritual inclinations before, she was unprepared for the effect it was going to have on her from the very beginning.

'I remember being in a friend's flat one day and he suggested we do a meditation together. I asked, "What's meditation?", and he just told me to lie down on the floor and that he would talk me through it.'

Linda lay down and experienced what she now calls an 'absolute connection' with something deep, something inexplicable, something that she still finds impossible to put into words.

'I was totally blown away. It was a complete "I've seen the light" kind of experience.'

For the remainder of her time in New York, she developed and kept up a strong meditation practice, seeking more of that intense experience of something beyond the known world.

Returning to Australia the following year and slotting back into her student life, her meditation practice became less important. By the time she had graduated, begun working and started studying for her Masters degree, the spiritual side of her nature had been all but forgotten.

In 2002, Linda was leading a busy life in the Melbourne beachside suburb of St Kilda. Her trendy one-bedroom apartment overlooked the ocean, where she enjoyed rollerblading every morning along the coastal paths. Halfway through her degree, she was already a practising psychologist and worked counselling students and staff at a city university institute. An active social life and strong connections to family and friends took up the rest of her time.

'I had a very supportive friendship group, which was really important to me. I was busy studying, busy working, busy with friends.'

One seemingly ordinary Tuesday morning, 28-year-old Linda arrived for work as usual and realised that her legs and feet had started to tingle and go numb. In fact, this had happened once before, exactly a year earlier, but despite her enquiring mind and her sister's medical background, it hadn't troubled her. The previous episode had been fairly mild, and although an MRI showed up one lesion on her spine, the diagnosis of transverse myelitis was delivered in the kind of reassuring manner that gave Linda no clue of what might be just around the corner. When those first symptoms resolved within six weeks as predicted, she believed the prognosis that there was nothing to worry about, and genuinely didn't give it another thought.

This recurrence in the spring of 2002 was immediately more concerning. The symptoms were spreading at an alarming rate, and from the start the numbness was far more intense. Linda went straight to her GP, who sent her to a neurologist for an MRI. By the time she arrived for the scan, the numbness had engulfed both her legs, and the next day when she returned for the results it had spread into her hands as well.

Sure enough, a second lesion was now apparent on her spinal cord and she was sent for intravenous steroid treatment. Surprisingly, the diagnosis of multiple sclerosis did not come straight away, and it was a chance comment from a young registrar in the hospital where Linda was receiving treatment that first alerted her to the possibility. While she was sitting in the waiting room the registrar appeared with a folder filled with medical notes. 'Oh, you're Linda, and you've got MS, right?' the registrar said.

'No, you've made a mistake, I've just got this numbness in my legs and hands,' replied Linda naively. That was the first time anyone had mentioned the disease.

Despite the steroid treatment, her symptoms continued to worsen. Within days she felt as though her chest was being clamped from the inside and it became difficult to breathe. By now both her legs were numb, tight, stiff and tingly right up to her buttocks, which felt like they had been permanently glued together. Her arms and hands were numb too, and she was struggling with nausea, dizziness and blurred vision.

'It was such a scary time,' Linda remembers. 'My whole body felt like it was not mine anymore.'

Clearly unable to stay alone in her flat, she was taken to the nearby home of her sister to be looked after by the extended family. Ani, her only sibling and fifteen years older than Linda, was already married with two teenage children. In the middle of Ani's lounge room was a large, soft, pastel-yellow sofa, where Linda was placed while different members of the family provided round-the-clock care, helping her into and out of bed, taking her to the toilet, cooking meals and even feeding her in the early days. Linda was weak, fatigued and in such a state of exhaustion and discomfort that she could barely raise her arms from her side. In the space of one week her busy life—professional, independent, active, fun—had crumbled around her, and she had been reduced to complete helplessness.

This was her physical situation when a second neurologist took one look at her, browsed through her notes and scans and gave the inevitable diagnosis of MS. This neurologist also gave Linda some options—not surprisingly, only medications. 'There are three drugs that may help,' he said. 'Go home and read through this literature, then come back and tell me which one you have decided to take.' It might seem that, at that stage, virtually immobile and needing 24-hour care, Linda was in no position to argue. But amazingly she felt a strong determination rise up within her, and she became completely convinced that drugs were not the answer for her—that there had to be another way out of this predicament. This came partly from a lifelong dislike of medication. But it also came from somewhere deep inside, from a place that was linked to her family's traumatic past.

Lying on the yellow couch in her sister Ani's house, Linda was unable to move and was totally dependent on her family for support. Her physical situation was extremely distressing. The clamping in her chest made every breath painful and difficult. Fatigue was so intense that lifting a pen was too much effort. Across the room, Linda could see a television in the corner. She wished she could watch something, but her blurred vision, dizziness and constant nausea made that impossible. Every time Linda needed to leave the couch—to go to the toilet, or to go to bed at the end of the day—it required a huge physical effort and assistance. Thankfully exhaustion was so great that sleep came fairly easily at night, though she had to keep her head propped up high to combat the dizziness. When she wore clothes at all they had to be very loose-fitting, and it was months before she could wear a bra.

She also had a problem with burning skin, caused by an extreme intolerance to heat. It was quite cool for November—unusual for Australia at that time of year—yet all the doors and windows were left open to try to accommodate Linda's heat sensitivity.

'I was lying on the couch, virtually naked, covered in wet sheets because my skin was just burning and that was the only thing that made a difference,' Linda remembers. 'But at the same time my skin was really painful to touch, so just having the sheets laid on top of me was almost unbearable.'

Lying in that state, unable to do anything for herself except breathe laboriously in and out, a kernel of recovery was starting to germinate. Linda began to turn inwards and reconnected with the two important lessons she had learned in New York—meditation and determination. This helped her through the weeks that followed.

'At first I was just meditating on breathing and being able to breathe more easily, and on getting some movement back, on practical physical things,' she says. Starting to see her illness as a wake-up call, Linda just lay there and listened to her body, waiting to see what would happen.

'I think that's where the strength came from,' she says. 'I had this real inner knowing that I was going to be okay, that despite everything I was going to be able to get through this.'

Linda's route to recovery required more than meditation and internal strength. It also required action. So she enlisted the help once again of her supportive family, who were always nearby. Ani, a medical doctor, and her parents were understandably concerned at Linda's decision to refuse pharmaceutical drugs. Nevertheless they accepted it and began sourcing other forms of healing that might fit with her chosen approach. Early on they discovered a holistic health practitioner in Melbourne, who recommended changing Linda's diet. With her Hungarian background, Linda had grown up as a carnivore, eating meat two if not three times a day. Cold cuts and pastrami for breakfast; bread, meat and cheese for lunch; meat and vegies for dinner. This was replaced with a very restricted diet consisting purely of vegetables, fish, nuts and seeds. No fruits or grains were allowed, nor any artificial or processed food of any kind. He also put her on a range of supplements.

'It was a big change from what I was used to, but in the scheme of things it was a small price to pay for potentially improving my health.'

More than six weeks passed, and every day Linda was helped onto the yellow couch. Across the room she could see through the big bay windows to the front yard, where two huge Moreton Bay fig trees took pride of place in front of the house. With her blurred vision, foggy thinking, clumsiness and forgetfulness, she wondered if she would ever be able to work or study again. Ani and her family carried on with their lives as best they could, but were very concerned about Linda's health. The phone rang often; Linda's friends wanted news of her condition, but visits were limited for fear of overwhelming her.

Linda stayed on the couch, meditating on her breathing, eating meals when they were brought, making assisted trips to the toilet. 'I'm sorry,' she would murmur as her sister took her weight yet again as she struggled to rise from the couch, 'I'm so sorry.' Always known for being strong and independent, like many people with MS, she was having a hard time adapting to being vulnerable.

The first sign of physical improvement came with Linda's breathing. One magical moment, instead of fighting pain and tightness with every inhalation, she began to breathe more easily. The relief she felt was enormous, and with it came a sense of tremendous gratitude and a real appreciation for every breath she took. A few days later her buttocks, which felt like they had been stuck together for weeks, came neurologically unglued. This was also a huge relief.

It was around this time that Ani, still searching for appropriate healing options for her sister, came across a copy of Professor George Jelinek's newly published first book, *Taking Control of Multiple Sclerosis.* She bought it and read it from cover to cover. She then started to share bits of it with Linda, who was still laid out on the sofa, experiencing fatigue, numbness, dizziness and blurred vision. Linda felt an immediate connection with the title of the book—'Taking Control'. That was what she had done as a child; taking control was something she was good at.

'When I listened to Ani reading the book, I remember feeling relieved that someone else had been through this and had found out all this information,' Linda reflects. 'I still felt incredibly unwell, but at the same time it was obvious to me that this was the right path, this is what I needed to follow, and I was really determined from the start.'

Linda stayed on her holistic doctor's diet for three months before switching to the Jelinek diet. This was an easy trade as she was then able to include fruit and grains in her meal plans, as well as the vegetables, fish, nuts, seeds and pulses she was already eating.

The weeks were passing incredibly slowly. Christmas came and went without a single photograph being taken to record the event.

Still unable to sit up vertically without being overcome with nausea and dizziness, Linda knew she couldn't return to her job. In fact it was a whole year before she felt well enough to take on that responsibility, though at the time she wasn't sure if she would ever work again. Her studies were a different matter. Most of the remaining work could be done from home and Linda started to entertain the idea of resuming her thesis at the start of the academic year in April 2003. She had also been planning to take a course on hypnotherapy, hoping to use it to supplement her clinical practice. She clung to this idea despite her illness, and with the help of a very caring and supportive teacher, Rob McNeilly, was able to enrol.

By March, Linda had recovered some movement in her body. Using the walls and furniture for support, she was able to walk short distances unaided. Fatigue was still a major problem, but the improvements in her physical situation meant she was able to leave her sister Ani's house and spend time with her Aunty Sue, who lived on the Mornington Peninsula coast, south of Melbourne. Linda had already spent some time with Sue when she first started on her new diet. 'Sue did the diet with me for the first couple of weeks,' she remembers. 'It was so helpful to have someone to support me through this significant lifestyle change—and someone to complain to when it got tough.'

Aunty Sue, her dad's sister, had become very significant in Linda's life since the death of her grandma the previous year. Right into adulthood, Linda had retained a feeling that when her grandma passed away, in a way her own life would also end, such was the connection she felt and the strength she drew from the relationship. She clearly remembers the night of her grandma's passing, seeing the events that unfolded as a strong spiritual sign.

'The night Grandma died the various members of our family had all been away and had just returned to Melbourne. My Aunty Sue—Grandma's daughter—was in town, and I had arranged to spend an evening with her for maybe only the second time in my adult life. We went for dinner together and had a lovely time.'

Later, back at the flat in St Kilda, Sue was about to leave for the night when Linda remembered a book she wanted to show her. Sue looked at the book for a while and was about to leave again when Linda remembered a photo album of her mother that she had made. Sue stayed to look at the photos. For the third time she put on her jacket and prepared to leave, this time getting as far as the front door when the phone rang. Linda interrupted their goodbyes to answer it. The call was from her father, giving the news that Grandma had just passed away.

'The fact that Aunty Sue was actually with me at that very moment that I had been dreading—the moment when I actually thought my own life might end—was very significant. It was like Grandma had orchestrated the whole thing, made sure there was someone to look out for me and handed the baton to Aunty Sue.'

Within minutes, the whole family had gathered at the deathbed. Linda remembers lying down beside her grandma's still-warm body.

'I just lay there on the bed and this completely white light enveloped us, and the most incredibly peaceful feeling came over me. It was a profound experience,' she says, 'a feeling that absolutely everything was going to be okay.'

Fittingly, the next step in Linda's recovery involved spending more time at Aunty Sue's house. It was there that her physical recovery really began. Able only to dress herself, go to the bathroom and shuffle short distances, at the start Linda's days were mainly spent resting and meditating on the balcony. Again a comfortable couch wasn't too far away whenever fatigue overwhelmed her. Parrots and honeyeaters came to visit the bird feeder, plant pots lined the timber railings, and through a row of tall trees she could just glimpse the ocean, with the waves crashing down on the beach.

After a few weeks, Linda's strength and mobility had improved enough for her to make her way very slowly down the single flight of stairs and into Sue's car. Then they drove the couple of hundred metres along a quiet road to the nearest beach access so that Linda could enjoy some exercise. These first tentative walks were very shaky, but it felt like freedom to be able to leave the couch after months of immobility. Whenever she walked, Linda gave herself a different marker to aim for: either a rock on the beach, or a signpost, or a tree—tiny signs of progress. Linda made the most of these first signs of physical improvement; she began to build yoga into her daily routine, gradually moving from simple poses to more challenging ones as her body allowed.

Meanwhile the hypnotherapy course had begun, and Linda was able to attend without too many modifications for her health. She started to incorporate the lessons from the course into her daily routine, and it had an immediate effect on her recovery.

Linda describes self-hypnosis as a form of meditation where you put your body and mind into a relaxed state and then suggest certain outcomes to yourself. These can be instructions to your body, desirable situations or general statements that you want to become true for you.

Quite early on after starting the course, Linda developed a mantra that she repeated to herself constantly throughout the day, and which she believes was important in her healing: 'Every cell in my body is healing every minute of every day.' Through self-hypnosis she also began to recognise how fatigue was affecting her, and found certain images very helpful. The first was the image of a sieve, as Linda realised that some people and situations were draining her of energy. She made it her business to find out where the energy was leaking from, and then find images to block the holes.

'These images were different every time,' says Linda. 'I used straw, glue or even concrete if the leak was really bad, to block the holes.'

A few months into the course, the numbness in Linda's arms had vanished and the tingling in her hands was decreasing. While celebrating the reduction in her symptoms, Linda did a very brave thing. Under self-hypnosis, she instructed her hands to tingle as a warning sign whenever she was pushing herself too hard physically, or becoming stressed by situations or relationships. This technique served Linda well over the years; she always found that her hands would be the first to let her know, before other symptoms spoke louder.

As her fitness gradually returned, Linda found she wanted to make the most of every moment in case these tastes of normal life were snatched away again.

'There was a constant balance between wanting to do everything immediately, but then stepping back so that I didn't overdo things. Finding this balance is a lifelong mission, though I am getting better at it,' she says.

In August 2003, Linda attended the second MS retreat ever held at The Gawler Foundation in Victoria's Yarra Valley, facilitated by Professor Jelinek. Linda spent much of the week resting on futons on the floor or lying on chairs during the sessions. She had come a long way since diagnosis, but her poor physical health still stood out among the group of people attending the retreat.

For Linda, the week represented another important step on her healing journey. With its emphasis on the mind–body connection, she describes it as a confronting yet nurturing experience, one in which she began to deal with emotional blockages from her past. It was here that she started to forgive her mother for leaving her at such a young age, work that she later continued through counselling.

After the retreat, Linda made a 'friends inventory' in which she listed the relationships that gave her energy and those that drained it.

'It may sound harsh, but I had to cull a couple of friends, and if a friendship was important to me but wasn't working then I addressed the issue. I became quite assertive,' she says. 'If people were supportive then great, but if not then friendships changed.'

By this time Linda had moved back into her own flat. Not quite ready for rollerblading yet, she was nevertheless able to shop, cook, clean and generally look after herself while continuing to complete her Masters degree and attend the hypnotherapy course one day a week. Her part-time job as a counsellor was still on hold until she felt strong enough, and cognitively and emotionally able to return. She was almost ready for that, but first she decided to fulfil a lifelong ambition and spend two months travelling in India with a friend. Her family was concerned, but once again Linda was determined. The trip, though hot and tiring, was successful and turned out to be a big confidence-booster for her.

Even so, it took a year of living alone before Linda felt a semblance of her former physical self, and there were lingering symptoms for a long time. She returned to her job as a psychologist and later moved into private practice, also running courses in relaxation and self-hypnosis. In time she began rollerblading again along the coastal paths, her long dark hair flowing behind her.

In her personal life, after the break-up of a significant long-term relationship just six weeks before her diagnosis, Linda had a few short-term relationships. Then in 2006 she met Tony, an Englishman who was on holiday in Melbourne. Linda describes him as compassionate, loyal, sincere, wise and understanding, just the kind of man who would have supported her through her illness—but in fact MS played no part in their lives.

They had a long-distance whirlwind romance, with Tony in London and Linda in Melbourne. For their third date they met up in Borneo—halfway between their two homes—and decided to climb Mount Kinabalu, the highest mountain in South-East Asia. Linda trained for it by running up and down the stairs of her apartment block, but she was very worried that fatigue might be a problem for her. When she and Tony reached the summit on the final day of the climb and saw the sunrise over the mountain, they had the feeling that together they could achieve anything. Eighteen months later they were married, and nine months after that their first child Joshua was born. MS seemed like a thing of the past.

Then in 2009, after they had been married for a couple of years and were living in central London, Linda came down with a really nasty dose of flu. Instead of bouncing back like normal after the virus, symptoms lingered and she began to feel her energy draining. Then she noticed her hands beginning to tingle and go numb. Terrified by what might be happening, she went to see a neurologist, who suggested she should have an MRI.

'I was really scared and I wasn't sure if I should do it or not—Tony had never seen me sick before. But I decided that knowledge is power, and at least if I had the MRI I would know where I stood.'

What could have been disaster ended up confirming Linda's recovery and bringing massive relief. Not only did the scan show that there were no new lesions in the last eight years, it also showed that the original lesions had disappeared.

'The report came back saying that one lesion had vanished completely, and the other was invisible to the naked eye and barely detectable, which was amazing.'

With medical proof to reassure her, Linda took the tingling and numbness in her hands as a warning sign from her body that she was doing too much.

'I eased off a bit and the symptoms went away. I think it was just my hands talking to me as I had asked them to,' she says.

It was then Linda realised that not only was recovery from MS possible, but that it had actually happened, and she had the confidence of knowing it was through her own efforts.

Linda Bloom still meditates and performs self-hypnosis most days. She has been relapse-free for ten years and has no MS symptoms whatsoever. A decade ago that would have seemed impossible, and

Linda keenly remembers the many lessons the illness has taught her.

'Being diagnosed with MS has been a huge blessing in my life and I am very grateful for it. It has helped me to re-evaluate what is important, understand my own unhelpful patterns, and make conscious decisions about how I want to live and contribute to the world,' she says.

Over the last two years, Linda has devoted much of her time to spreading the message of holistic healing for people with MS. This voluntary work fits in around her growing family; she and Tony celebrated the birth of baby Ella in August 2012.

'I strongly believe that the mind and body have incredible healing potential,' Linda reflects. 'Within us all there is strength, resilience and amazing power. When they are harnessed, anything is possible.'

RECOVERY

Recovery after a diagnosis of multiple sclerosis is possible. Our dozen examples bear witness to that fact. That doesn't mean that recovery is the same for everyone; similarly, as recovery and MS haven't really been associated in the past, what actually constitutes recovery remains a matter of some debate and discussion.

Has Wendy recovered, for example? She still has disability, her balance isn't good at times, and her mobility could be better. But we would argue that recovery is a gradual process, and that Wendy is well advanced along it. She has successfully reversed her physical and mental decline and is now clearly enjoying very noticeable and lasting improvements to her health. There is no doubt the illness has stabilised and that she is steadily regaining abilities and function she thought were lost forever. Her life is positive now, and she gets great enjoyment from things she thought she might never do again. Importantly, she has been able to maintain the goals and dreams she had prior to the diagnosis of MS.

Has Phil recovered? He finds he still throws his right foot a bit after a strenuous six kilometre (three and three-quarter mile) walk, but at 67 years old, many of his friends without MS are struggling to keep up! Most of his symptoms—ones that were completely debilitating a few years ago—have now gone. He no longer limps, his activities are not limited by the illness, his life is rich and full. An eighteen-hole round of the golf course is simply no problem anymore; it is just good fun, as it is supposed to be.

Wendy is recovering, Phil is recovering, and so are all the people in this book—and, of course, the authors. This is in sharp contrast with the prevailing paradigm of the illness, and of its historical context. People simply did not recover from MS; while some authorities talk about benign MS, we know from the research findings that people with this form of the illness—so-called 'benign' because people did not seem to deteriorate over time—did just that. While their progression to disability was slower than average, they *did* progressively get worse, often subtly, over time. This is not happening to the people in this book. Recovery is a real thing for them, with tangible permanent changes in how they feel and function, with positive spin-offs in their enjoyment of life and living. They are not getting worse, they are getting better.

While recovery means and entails different things to different people, it has some common features. Our participants in general demonstrate major transformations of their lives, in all sorts of ways. Megan struggled to find any triggers for the disease when confronted with that question. But with application and hard work, she began to see the emotional cost of putting a brave face on everything, for everybody. And once she became aware of the underlying issues, her life was transformed; she was able to live a more authentic life, true to herself. Of course, many of our friends and relatives are much more comfortable with us staying as we are, and feel threatened by such transformation—the end result of which can be significant changes to our relationships, as in Megan's case.

The priming effect of hope seems a universal first step to recovery. Faith that gradually gives way to belief can then follow, faith in oneself and one's future. A curiosity about and willingness to explore difficult issues, and understand the meaning of the illness, also seem important. For many of our participants, meditation has been a significant aspect of this part of the journey. And, of course, courage, determination and a willingness to embrace change also form important components of recovery.

A key defining feature of recovery, though, is that it requires action. It necessitates doing something. Recovery doesn't just happen; all our survivors are characterised by the action they took, the changes they made, the path they followed, what they did to get better. None was a passive victim. And for many, doing something about the diagnosis of MS involved some risk—it wasn't a comfortable process. Several had to make complex internal changes that required great courage, facing enormous and sometimes long-standing fears. But all of them found that they also had to change some relatively simple lifelong habits to get well.

Changing habits and lifestyle is an active process; it is not a passive one. Interestingly, though, habits are just that—habits. Once people make changes to bad habits and develop good habits, the good habits are just as hard to change as the bad ones were. That is one of the reasons we advocate an 'all-or-nothing' approach. We might as well, for example, give up all meat, rather than continue having a small piece of chicken breast once a week. Placing a particular food item on a pedestal, as it were, affords it 'treat' status, whether it be occasional meat, or chocolate, or any other food that is damaging to our health, but perceived as highly desirable. Hanging on to the old habit means that one never really adopts the new one. Once the new habit of not eating meat is in place, it is just as hard to break as the old habit of eating meat. The same applies to many of the lifestyle choices our survivors have made in order to recover. As Phil found out, it pays to be really rigorous in changing lifestyle habits if one is to fully regain health.

THE ADVANTAGES OF SERIOUS ILLNESS

Interestingly, some people who recover from MS, and other serious illness, come to see distinct advantages to having had the disease. Some see it as providing a reason to undertake inner journeys they had not felt brave enough to confront without the diagnosis. Not only does the illness provide a reason to start eating well and avoid those common foods and other things that are toxic in our environment, many feel it legitimises the exploration of spiritual and emotional issues that may have gone unexplored without the diagnosis.

For some, serious illness is like a loud knock at the door of life. Many have heard muffled scratchings at the door before, and been vaguely aware that something wasn't right, but a life-changing diagnosis puts the 'dis-ease' in life—the imbalance and lack of ease—squarely in one's face. While denial works for some, for a while and only to a limited extent, if recovery is going to be a possibility there is no hiding from the diagnosis. It simply has to be dealt with.

And dealing with longstanding issues that rob us of our energy is liberating. We get our energy back. There is little doubt that the enormous sense of relief we get when we finally face and sort out difficult issues is extremely healing for our bodies, as well as our minds. Gaspar losing his need for perfection, Megan dropping her brave face, Linda letting go of her resentment towards her mother: there is a clear sense from their stories that these issues needed resolution before physical health was possible. And so it has transpired.

Embarking on the road to recovery from MS is an enormous journey, involving so many changes and so much courage. In their own ways, each of our participants has demonstrated the breadth of the task with which they were confronted, and the faith and courage they needed to overcome MS.

FINDING HOPE

But they all had to start with hope. Hope is the first and most basic ingredient of recovery. Without hope, in the midst of despair, it is impossible even to take the first step, to know the direction in which to head. All of our participants found hope, and that gave them the necessary energy to start the journey to recovery.

This is one of the biggest problems with much of the modern management of MS. Adopting a drug-only approach to managing the illness is essentially negative. Put simply, it says that the drugs will slow things down, at some cost, but they offer no hope of actually regaining good health. They just slow things down, and for many of the drugs not even by much. If that is all that is offered, deep down, most people realise on reflection that the outlook remains rather negative. They have to comply with instructions and take the medication daily, or second daily, or weekly, or monthly, and anticipate negative side effects, possibly with blood testing along the way, only to look forward to a less precipitous decline.

This isn't real hope.

Drugs can form part of a bigger package that does offer the genuine prospect of actually getting better. In that sense, they can be part of a strategy that offers hope, and allows people to use their own efforts to regain their health. Allowing people with MS to feel they have some control, while at the same time using medication to assist in gaining some physical stability with the illness, empowers people, enabling them to be in charge of their own health. Of course, many will opt to pursue genuine health without taking any of the medications, as a number of our survivors have.

But the hope needs to be credible. It needs to be built on a solid foundation; it needs to be real. We can all spot lack of credibility and authenticity. Hope that is based on wishful thinking, and positivity without foundation, get us nowhere, because we soon find out that they don't actually work. This disease can be relentless and ruthless if we don't really confront it, and it becomes obvious very quickly to most people if it is progressing. To start the process of confronting the illness, we need real hope. Fortunately, there is now a solid science behind the role that environmental factors play in increasing the risk of progression of MS, in a very similar way to the deterioration from other more common Western diseases.

We now have solid evidence, for example, that coronary heart disease, long thought to be only manageable with drugs and surgery, can actually be reversed with a multi-dimensional approach, similar to the *Overcoming Multiple Sclerosis* approach. Prostate cancer too can be successfully treated, with regression of the cancer, with the same approach. We have US physician Dr Dean Ornish to thank for these breakthroughs, and his programs are now Medicare-funded and being rolled out across American hospitals.

Our own data indicate that this approach is now bearing fruit for people with MS; our publications show that people attending residential retreats to learn how to live this way are on average 20 per cent better after five years. Now that is real hope! The disease hasn't just stabilised once the modifiable risk factors are attended to: people actually get better, many of them recovering, just as our participants in this book have.

So real hope is a vital first ingredient before the illness can be dealt with. Real hope leads to a sense of positivity and empowerment—that it is actually possible to make a difference to one's health, even in the face of what is generally thought to be an incurable, progressively disabling condition, through one's own efforts. This is an enormously empowering position, and one that is vastly different from being the passive recipient of drug therapy and disability supports, as well-intentioned as these interventions might be. Look at Carrie's story: predictions of doom and gloom, and nothing positive to hang on to led her to gradually get depressed. Then hope arrived, and suddenly she found some energy and positivity, and she was able to do something about her situation.

The positivity that is generated from being in this position is real. It is not just putting a brave face on a difficult situation, or wishful thinking. People who really accept that it is possible to change the course of this illness live life differently because of their positivity. This is reflected in their quality of life—that is how living their lives actually feels to them. Our data demonstrate this very dramatic improvement in the quality of life for people living this way.

To begin with, though, after finding hope it is necessary to have some faith that this will work. We see faith as the process where one lives as if the desired outcome will be what actually comes to pass. That is, it is not necessary to believe that one will recover, but to live as if that will happen. Belief can come later, when time has passed, and things start to improve, and health stabilises. Rebecca's story illustrates this well—the gradual cementing of belief as her health continued to improve. Living without this faith, and being at the mercy of fear of the future, is a very energy-sapping process, and is really not conducive to recovery. From the kernel of hope, fostered by this faith in oneself and the future, genuine belief that recovery is possible can grow.

Hope and faith also lead to the realisation that a person diagnosed with MS has choices. Initially, after diagnosis, things look bleak for most people, as a future of disability and dependence seems the only possible outcome. But the hope of a different outcome, together with credible information supporting this possibility, leads to an appreciation that actually, a person diagnosed with MS has many choices, and there are many possible outcomes. Initially, choices about food, exercise, stress reduction, supplements and so on. But with time, further choices about how to live one's life, the friends one chooses, relationships, work.

The sense of having choices is also empowering.

SPIRITUALITY AND THE DIFFICULT QUESTIONS

One of the most obvious choices is how to respond to the illness. This may not seem a choice at first, until one has some hope. Some people respond to the diagnosis of serious illness with denial. While denial is an effective tool in the short term for reducing pain and suffering, in the longer term it doesn't work, because there is no engagement with the illness and the issues it raises. For many people, and all the people in this book, the diagnosis of serious illness presents a choice about one's engagement with life. For many, it demands confronting the big questions in life. What is the purpose of my life? How am I living my life? What does my life mean? Why am I here? What about death, what does that mean?

For most people, really effectively dealing with an illness demands that one addresses a whole range of emotional, psychological and spiritual issues, as well as the more commonly discussed physical issues like nutrition, exercise, stress reduction and so on. The stark reality of facing what most authorities agree is a steady loss of function and ability—often well before reaching any kind of older age—is enormously confronting, and throws these and many other questions up. They are not trivial questions and they demand to be dealt with. And for many people, given that MS often strikes at a young age, it may be the first time they have ever seriously considered such things.

So to really have any chance of recovering, the approach has to be multi-dimensional, and for most people includes a deeper exploration of meaning and purpose in life. Gaspar, lying in his hospital bed, chose to look up at what was important in life, and in an instant he felt peace. Jack's faith sustained him in his recovery. Megan actually had to unravel her life to find what was wrong and reinvent herself, getting back in the driver's seat of her own life, with her own purpose and authenticity driving her, rather than others' expectations. Linda saw clear spiritual signs as she gradually recovered physically, and used the experience to help her decide what was important in her life, how she wanted to live and, above all, give her a clearer sense of how she might contribute, and of her life's meaning. A chance radio broadcast provided Wendy with the glimmer of hope to start a process that culminated in her reflecting on her life, unlocking years of grief in a flood of tears, and confronting long-held emotional repression and unfinished business.

Recovery for our dozen people has not been just about physical changes; we would argue that confronting the 'dis-ease' in one's life—looking at how one is living life, and examining the big, important questions—is a key component.

MEDITATION

One of the tools that makes this journey easier for many people is meditation. Meditation has been around as a healing and spiritual practice for thousands of years. And it has a proven track record. Typing 'meditation' into PubMed—the National Library of Medicine's bibliographic database of papers published in the world's leading medical journals—results in over 2500 citations. Interestingly, there was a peak in these publications in the 1970s, particularly around transcendental meditation, then things went quiet until around the turn of the millennium, probably reflecting that period in the West where there was generally thought to be a concentration on material things, and a lack of spirituality. Since then, there has been a steady increase in publications, peaking with 240 in 2011—mostly now about mindfulness meditation.

The health benefits of meditation are now well accepted by medical researchers. What is not so well studied or understood is the spiritual benefit. A regular practice of meditation brings not only health benefits, with an alteration of our response to life stresses, but peace of mind, so that we can handle our changing outer life circumstances with inner equanimity and calm. But meditation also allows us to more deeply engage with life's difficult questions, and find our own unique answers to what provides us with meaning. Recovering from MS may be possible without such engagement, but the experience of most of our survivors suggests it is easier with it.

COURAGE AND DETERMINATION

Confronting difficulty, engaging with life, and living an authentic life actually all require a good deal of courage. Denial does not.

Despite being a courageous and determined person—as Carrie had to be in juggling the demands of motherhood, being a breadwinner, and a very demanding job with unsociable hours—denial left Carrie in a passive, negative place, allowing worries about the future and her health to dominate her life, while MS continued its steady progression in the background. Her longstanding determination was being used to get her through each day, but it wasn't really directed at her own health, her own future. Turning that determination and courage towards positive action directed at recovery actually turned her life around. It actually gave her the energy ultimately to continue with life on her terms, and even to start giving back to the community by volunteering and helping others find their own solutions, as others in our group of survivors have done.

It is courageous to embark on a whole new way of living, changing diet and lifestyle dramatically, slipping out of the comfortable role that friends and relatives have you slotted into. It is risky business. People are often frightened of change; staying the same as you have always been is very reassuring to most people around us, partners and loved ones included. Challenging such relationships and friendships, however, may be necessary if recovery is to become more than a possibility—if recovery is to become a reality. One can find that friends disappear—even friends you may have thought were there for the long haul—once you start making big changes. Linda came to realise that certain people in her life were draining away the energy she needed if she was to heal, and she made conscious decisions about who was to remain in her circle of friends; and she finally found the supportive partner she needed.

It is courageous to explore one's longstanding emotional difficulties, to spend time working through relationship issues—sometimes culminating in leaving those relationships, as some of our survivors have discovered. Relationships that seemed stable can founder, once one half of the relationship makes decisions that threaten its stability. Megan discovered such an issue, and had to find the courage to end her marriage—a decision she regarded as utterly selfish, yet one she simply knew she had to make.

However, many people feel the response and support of their loved ones are a crucial component of recovery. Many of our survivors found their relationships improved once they started making changes. They took a risk, and they were rewarded with more understanding, better friendship, and a deeper connection with their loved ones. Gaspar appeared to be more present, more there for his partner, even while lying immobile in a hospital bed. Sam's recovery noticeably improved his relationships, both with family and his wife-to-be, Lisette. Jack and Silvia enjoyed sharing his little outbursts of enthusiasm as hope turned to recovery. Keryn and Linda were both rewarded for taking risks and making changes in finding love and support from those closest to them, and partners who understood and valued their journeys.

The feeling that one is not alone and isolated, that one can depend on others, can be connected with a group of like-minded people, appears important to recovery. Many of our survivors attended live-in week-long retreats to kick-start their recoveries. While total immersion in everything that one can do about MS is part of the goal of these retreats, another important aspect is the close bonding that occurs—the natural sharing of innermost feelings, anxieties and emotions. Having the courage to attend a retreat, and to open up in a group of 30–40 people, has an amazing effect in breaking down barriers between people, but also in generating lifelong friendships and support. The groups often keep in touch through social media or in person at reunions, or small get-togethers. The love, compassion and support they generate are pivotal in generating the necessary emotional stability for healing and recovery.

TRANSFORMATION

Recovery is an odd word in one sense. The 're-' part suggests some going back or returning to some previous state. None of our twelve survivors, however, is the same today as when first diagnosed; each of them has irrevocably changed, and none of them would revoke that change. Gaspar and Sam have been told by their neurologists that it is no longer possible to make a diagnosis of MS, Sam even having the original diagnosis questioned. They have essentially been told they no longer have MS. Yet, neither of them would change back to who they were and how they lived prior to diagnosis, and nor would any of the others. Recovery requires transformation; recovery *is* transformation.

All of our MS survivors are transformed, physically, and often emotionally or spiritually as well. They are different people than when they began their journeys. Surprisingly, perhaps, many express gratitude for the opportunity this serious illness has given them to transform their lives. But none of them used the word 'recovery' in our interviews. Perhaps for fear of jinxing their futures, of tempting fate. Or for some of them, perhaps their faith hasn't yet turned to belief. Or they just didn't like the word, or the concept. Or they are tempted at times to believe the sceptics who say that MS is so unpredictable.

But looking on, from a distance, it is easier for us. In looking up definitions of the word 'recovery' we came across 'restoration to a former or better condition', highlighting this issue of a return to a previous state. But what we have seen is that all of these survivors have found a *better* condition. They are in a place they would rather be now, and we're convinced they have recovered; they are so enormously transformed that actually MS no longer has any serious currency in their lives. They are different, they feel different, they live differently, and have no intention of returning to how they previously lived.

And their fear of MS, their fear of the future, has evaporated.

FACING FEAR

Fear is destructive. Look at Keryn's early experience after diagnosis. She was literally terrified—terrified of what was happening to her, terrified of the future. Her fear was so tangible that it paralysed her, left her feeling that there was nothing she could do. Remaining in that place, consumed by fear, paralysed and unable to move in any direction, is how depression starts, as it did for Carrie and Ginny. It is an enormously passive position, feeling that one is essentially at the mercy of a disease that will run its own course, and rob one of strength and feeling.

It is interesting to look at the metaphor here. Many people when they describe fear talk about feeling paralysed, feeling numb with fear. And these are exactly the physical effects that MS causes. Fear clearly has a very negative synergistic effect on MS, making the disease, and life for the person, worse. We now have quite good data to show that people with MS who have been consumed by fear, who are depressed, literally have more of the chemicals in their bodies that are associated with inflammation than those who are not depressed. Inflammation is the core disease process in MS. This is more than just theoretical, or a way of framing the illness. Fear drags one down, metaphorically and literally.

So if fear is such a negative influence for people with MS, what should be done about it? Our survivors' experience is that hope is the necessary first ingredient, and in the longer term the antidote to fear is faith—to live life as if things will turn out the way we plan them to. It also helps to confront one's fears, and explore them before they can really be let go. Look at Craig: the moment the story of his difficulties and fears came pouring out to Janine, he sowed the seeds of his recovery. When Gaspar began to replace his fears of a dependent future with images of joy and beauty, he began to have faith, and his life began to change. Jack, hearing 'Healer' on his iPod, felt his fears melt and he knew that he would be okay. Rebecca was consumed by fear initially, and this worsened as her condition deteriorated; then the spark of hope appeared when she found Dr Roy Swank's paper on the web, and for the first time she felt some energy return, and she knew there was something she could do.

Generally, our survivors knew intuitively that they could not remain in a state of fear—that fear would ultimately paralyse them. And through hope, and gradually through faith, they overcame their fears, and began their roads to recovery.

RIDE ON FEARLESSLY

What we wish is that we could bring this simple message of hope to everyone in the world with MS, and as soon as possible after diagnosis. The enormity of the grief that follows MS diagnosis, experienced by everyone who understands what the diagnosis has always been considered to mean, need no longer be endured. As well as sound scientific evidence that MS can be controlled and indeed overcome, and group data showing improvement for those making significant lifestyle changes, we now have the human experience that validates the science.

These are real people, and they have really recovered. With all their human frailties, fears and anxieties, their longings and their searching, they have found answers where we have never really thought answers were possible. We hope that the intimate close-ups of their lives that we have presented will give others with MS, and those close to people with MS, the confidence that this really is possible—that recovering from multiple sclerosis is not wishful thinking.

Looking at these people and their stories, it becomes obvious that one doesn't need to be some kind of super-hero to recover. Ordinary people can recover, and this is possible even after many years with the illness, even with progressive MS. It is also obvious that recovery can involve many different paths, and involves different things for different people. The road to recovery probably reflects the type of person involved, and what is important to them. For Ginny and Rebecca it was about intellectually satisfying themselves of the science behind the various diet and lifestyle recommendations they researched; for Linda, Gaspar and others, the spiritual journey was a key component. But for all of them, it took courage, and persistence, and a very significant commitment and determination. But when faced with the prospect of steady deterioration, mentally and physically, why wouldn't one commit to it? What did they have to lose?

People diagnosed with MS stand at a major crossroads in their lives; for many it will be the most important crossroads they encounter. They have choices, although this may not be immediately obvious, and the choices they make will determine where they find themselves decades later. Every seemingly simple inconsequential choice today determines our health tomorrow. Everything matters.

The future is far more in our hands than we are led to believe by our medical advisers.

A commitment to do whatever it takes to get well, to undertake a serious examination of one's life, both internal and external, to ride on fearlessly—that is the common theme of the dozen MS survivors in this book. Recovery from MS did not happen to any of these people by accident; recovery rarely does. Aiming for recovery is not by any means an easy road, but the rewards are clear. A new life awaits those prepared to embark on this journey—an authentic, transformed life. Now, isn't that a prize worth aiming for?

From the two of us, George and Karen, and the twelve survivors who have shared their stories here, we wish you clarity in your choices, and the strength and courage to face your fears. We wish you long, healthy and happy lives, full of peace and joy; we hope your journeys towards recovery will be rich, exciting and fulfilling.

Be well.

BACK COVER MATERIAL

'THIS IS A MUST READ FOR ANYONE WITH MS. RECOVERY IS ACHIEVABLE. IT IS ALL ABOUT THE LIFESTYLE CHOICES WE MAKE EVERY DAY!'

Dr Terry Wahls, MD, author of *Minding My Mitochondria*

A diagnosis of multiple sclerosis conjures up images of wheelchairs and a shortened life, but in fact it's possible to regain mobility and make a recovery. These deeply moving life stories of twelve people from around the world offer real hope to people with MS everywhere. These determined women and men have been able to halt the progression of the disease and recover mobility by making significant lifestyle changes including diet, sunshine, meditation, exercise, and for some, using drug therapy.

Based on extended interviews, these stories offer an insight into the different journeys to recovery. They also highlight the challenges faced by people with different types of MS and at different stages in the progression of the disease.

PROFESSOR GEORGE JELINEK is author of the internationally successful guide *Overcoming Multiple Sclerosis.* Diagnosed with MS in 1999, he is symptom free. He is an academic emergen-

cy physician at the University of Melbourne and Monash University, Australia.

KAREN LAW is a journalist who has worked in the UK and Australia and is recovering from MS.

Printed in Great Britain
by Amazon

62531610R00165